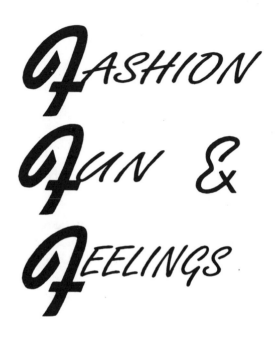

*F*ASHION
*F*UN &
*F*EELINGS

A Lady's Perspective on Fashion and Life

By T. J. Reid

Christmas 2017 With my love!

FASHION, FUN & FEELINGS

A Lady's Perspective on Fashion and Life

By T. J. Reid

Published by:
Retail Resources Publications
P.O. Box 977
403 N. Duncan Avenue
Amite, Louisiana 70422

First Edition

Copyright © 1993 by T. J. Reid

Printed in the United States of America

ISBN: 1-880522-48-9

Library of Congress Catalog Card Number: 83-93566

Book Production and Cover Design by ONE-ON-ONE BOOK DESIGN, West Hills, California

Front cover photo by Kate Lightfoot, FASHION CONNECTION, Hammond, Louisiana

Printed by Century Graphics Corporation, Metairie, Louisiana

DEDICATION

When I first began writing this book several years ago, I decided it would be dedicated to all the women who had influenced my life. After I started the list, I realized I had a perfect ten, and perhaps should borrow a trick or two from David Lettermen and call it my own TOP TEN WOMEN I OWE MY LIFE TO.

Of course, I'd begin with my grandmother JoJo, in memory of all her teachings that have lasted me a lifetime; then I'd mention Mother, but not much since she's already had one whole book dedicated to her. Aunt Sugar needs a world of thanks for always being there when I needed a Godmother and all the other roles she filled in my life. I need to thank my mother-in-law Dottie, for never being a mother-in-law, just being a wonderful loving friend, and Larry's grandmother, Meme, was my example of what a Southern lady should be. The center of my feminine universe is my only daughter, Laura Lea, today's generation of the Reid woman. She's so strong, so feisty, yet so kind and gentle, and PERFECT in her mother's eyes.

My mentor in this new career of image, speaking, and writing deserves a salute. I'll always remember the afternoon Gail Florin spent forcing me to repeat en-tre-per-nu-er until I finally pronounced it right.

The person who furnishes the glue to hold me together is Marsha. She's there every day, not just as an assistant, not just as a sister-in-law, but as caretaker and friend. She's played nurse, driver, and helper as much as my Kim, who moved to Florida and broke my heart by being so far away. Our time together is very limited now, but she's always in my heart, and on my phone bill.

And then there's my Aunt Cordelia, who brags about me to total strangers on the street, (you may have met her, she carries my book and tape around with her at the grocery store), and all my favorite female cousins, too many to count.

In everyone's life there's a friend: that one person who knows, who cares, who understands, and who never judges, just accepts. I may go days without a word, or see her for hours on end, but forever Betty is with me. If ever God gave me a sister, a partner, a person who matters—it's Betty, and for that I feel blessed.

So, to whom is this book dedicated? I'm not really sure, but I think I lost count and messed up THE TOP TEN theory. What's this book about? Women—their fashions, their fun, and their feelings!

Therefore, after giving it more thought, I dedicate this book to TOM CRUISE.

Read on, you'll understand!

ACKNOWLEDGMENTS

Special permission was given by THE MERIDIAN CORPORATION for references from *Your Ideal Silhouette* by Gail Florin.

Special appreciation to Sally Horner, President of IMAGE INTERNATIONAL for permission to reprint portions from her book, *Earrings That Enhance*. Sally is a speaker/consultant from Erie, Pennsylvania.

Some of the chapters in the section FEELINGS were previously printed in *The News Digest*, Amite, Louisiana, under the byline of "A Woman's Place" by T. J. Reid.

A sincere thanks to Carolyn Porter of ONE-ON-ONE BOOK PRODUCTION for being the lady who helped put all the pieces together.

My appreciation to THE DALLAS APPAREL MART, Dan Bruce, Debbie Francis, Beth Gorman, and the QVC CABLE NETWORK for giving me the opportunity to begin a new career, and achieve a dream.

ABOUT THE AUTHOR

T.J. Reid describes herself as one of the first of the Baby Boomer generation—a daughter, a wife, a mother, and a full-time career woman. In *FASHION, FUN, AND FEELINGS* she combined all these job descriptions into one, blending her talents and expertise as a nationally acclaimed fashion/accessory authority with the humor, happiness, and heartache of the Southern belle she proudly confesses to be.

A fashion retailer for over twenty years, T. J. gave up a very successful business career in mid-life to become a consultant, professional speaker, author, and television personality. She truly exemplifies the quote, "We must give up who we are for what we can become." (She's living proof, it works!)

Growing up as an only child, in a small Louisiana community of less than 3,000 people, T. J. dreamed of becoming a fashion designer, a best selling writer, a movie star, or just simply moving far, far away to the big city! She succeeded in making it fifteen miles down the road to a rural Southern community of almost 5,000 people where she shares her life with husband, Larry, and a one-eyed cat called "Cootie." You'll meet her two grown children: Billy and Laura Lea, on the pages of this book, along with the many friends and foes who make up this fun-filled story.

T. J.'s theory of life is that YOU CAN HAVE IT ALL, and through these chapters, she relates the excitement, emotion, and energy she uses to live and dress each day to the fullest because LIFE IS NO DRESS REHEARSAL!

Table of Contents

SECTION III—FEELINGS

INTRODUCTION

I wrote FASHION, FUN, AND FEELINGS for many reasons. The Fashion section started out as a way to answer all the women who constantly ask me about their wardrobe problems. None of these are ever life shattering decisions, but simply little how-to questions that they would like answered by someone they consider a "fashion consultant."

Each time I complete a seminar or presentation, there is never enough time for each attendee to have their turn, but I've noticed no matter where I am, Montana or Mississippi, New York or New Mexico, the same questions are asked. If I receive letters following a television appearance, the same topics are addressed. After all, there are just so many ways to wear a garment, tie a scarf, or select a handbag.

It didn't take long to realize one book could solve all these problems, answer all the basic questions, and still have lots of pages left over! Seeing the blank sheets, I decided to use the space to tell women what I consider the priorities of life—not as a fashion authority, but as a WOMAN. I wanted to touch on style, love, and laughter. I decided to share what I know about skirt lengths, scarf tying, and hosiery colors, but also what I feel about caring, understanding, kindness, compassion, and friendship.

No, I'm not a shrink, a medical doctor, or any other educated expert with initials behind my name. (Although the *California Apparel News* did once call me "America's fashion therapist.")

I am just a woman, which fills all the qualifications of being an authority on this topic. I am a daughter, a wife, a mother, a daughter-in-law, a friend, a professional speaker, a business executive, a fashion journalist, an author, a Democrat, a Christian, a Southerner, a Taurus, and according to Carole Jackson's *Color Me Beautiful* theory: a dramatic winter. That sure sounds like enough credentials to me!

I speak with authority when I say, "No bare legs with a business ensemble," but I speak with heart when I say "Live each day as if it were your last." A woman's life should never revolve around what she has on today, but rather how she feels about waking up. It's wonderful if your nail polish matches your outfit, but God only cares what your hands are doing—not what they're wearing. Your lips can be lovely in perfect pink lipstick, but the words which pass across them are what truly counts. Hats are glamorous, but it's what's inside your head that matters most, not what's sitting on it!

As you read through the three sections of this book, keep this thought in mind:

WHEN YOU START OUT THE DOOR EACH MORNING TO FACE THE WORLD, THE MOST IMPORTANT THING TO WEAR IS A S-M-I-L-E!

SECTION I

FASHION

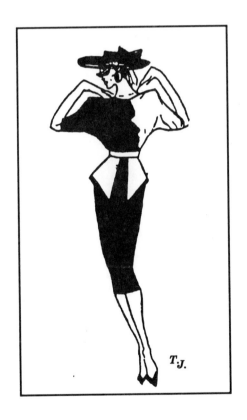

Head-to-Toe Terrific!

What a wonderful compliment! Every woman I know would like to have this term used to describe the way she looks, whether eighteen or eighty. These fashion chapters were written to help you hear these words! (That's a promise.) I can't swear to create a brand new you in two weeks, or inspire you to lose fifty pounds in two months, or help you win Miss America this year (unless you are already MISS TEXAS), BUT if you follow the advice on these pages, you'll definitely find new, exciting, and affordable ways to look better than you ever imagined possible.

This is not a self-help change-your-life make-over, but a how to create the best YOU, you can be. Learn how to accentuate your positives, cover up your negatives, and enjoy each tomorrow by saving yourself time, money, and mental anguish!

It has been said, "One picture is worth a thousand words," so rather than taking up more space with unnecessary syllables, I invite you to turn the page and see for yourself...

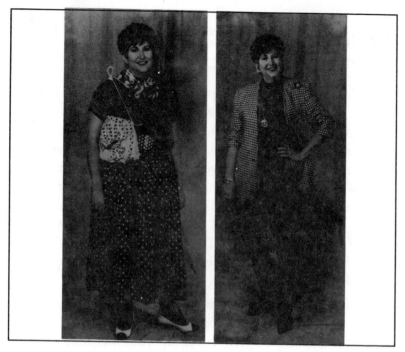

This is T.J. (me) **BEFORE,** and this is T.J. (me, again) **AFTER.**

No, I didn't go on a diet, have surgery, or use a doctored photograph. These pictures were taken five minutes apart, and if you notice—nothing changed excepted my clothing and accessories.

The lipstick, the hair, the make-up, even my smile is the same. Unlike those before-after shots usually used to show how much better a person looks after one of those miracle diet plans, I purposely chose not to alter my facial expression. I was smiling each time BUT ...in the after, I have something to SMILE about. I've visually lost over 25 pounds just by using the principles discussed in the following pages.

Now that I have your attention, read on. See how easy it is to achieve the same fashion success without giving up dessert!

Four

HATS—THE EXCITING ACCESSORY

WHEN/WHAT/HOW/WHERE/WHY

WHEN: A hat dramatizes you and what you wear. It adds zest to any outfit, so wear a hat for style, wear a hat for fun, and wear a hat for a feminine finished, complete look.

WHERE: A hat is appropriate at poolside, on the beach, when gardening, for walking, for working, at luncheons and teas, to church, to corporate meetings and seminars, at daytime weddings, at garden parties, for cocktails, and for dining out.

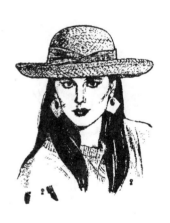

HOW: DO NOT wear a hat on the back of your head. For current fashion it looks awkward and unstylish. A hat loses it's charm and importance if worn incorrectly. Most hats are best worn pulled down well on the head over the forehead towards the eyes.

WHAT: Since a hat makes a definite fashion statement, almost everything you wear looks better with one!

❋ Big brims look good with sundresses for the beach or poolside. Sexy for soft breeezy fabrics and elegant with satins and ribbons. Try a floppy wide brim.

❋ Sailors, fedoras, and bowlers are ideal with suits. Dress 'em up or down for a fashion or a fun touch; be serious or silly—it's your choice.

Five

✳ Cowboy hats, French berets, Italian fedoras, and the All-American baseball cap cover an international line-up of toppings for jeans and casual wear. Add glitter, glitz, and jewels for more excitement.

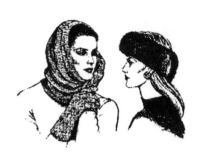

✳ Toques, turbans, and pill-boxes (a la Jackie O.) compliment a coat or fur.

✳ Profile styles and wide brims are perfect for dress.

✳ Mini-caps, shells, turbans, and even decorated veils go to dinner and make evenings elegant.

Wearing a hat lends an air of importance, sophistication, mystery, innocence, and let's not forget—sexiness! Men stop in their tracks for ladies in hats. They love 'em, and respect them (remember their grand-mothers and mothers WORE hats!).

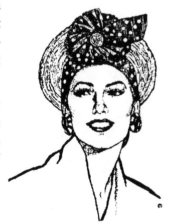

Wearing a hat will boost your confidence (or at least make you appear "all together" to the rest of the world). Set yourself apart from the rest. Make a personal fashion statement. Be well-hatted, USE YOUR HEAD!

I am a lady who loves hats. I enjoy the feeling of self-confidence that automatically comes with wearing a hat. It portrays a woman with a positive attitude who knows who she is and where she's going. FRANK OLIVE, millinery designer, named one of America's 100 most influential fashion creators of the century by *Women's Wear Daily*, puts it this way, "A hat

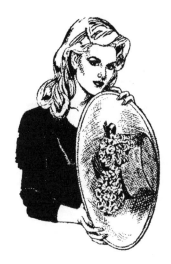

transforms any woman into an exciting personality with a sense of drama. A hat adds a third dimension to its wearer—intimidating, captivating, allowing her to reveal or veil her innermost thoughts and emotions. It casts an aura of mystery, of authority and dignity, sometimes a hint of flirtatiousness. Simply stated, a hat is magic!"

He suggests a woman needs to stand in front of a full-length mirror, holding a hand mirror to reflect different angles. This is the only true way to completely see the hat you are trying on. To select the appropriate style, please consider:

- the neckline
- the shape of the shoulder
- the length of the skirt
- the shape of the shoe and height of the heel
- the color and texture of the outfit
- the overall silhouette and complete look

EARRINGS — WHY BOTHER?

Would you have a photo on the wall without a frame? Would you bake a birthday cake and not add icing? Would you wrap a gift without a ribbon or a bow? Of course not!

So think of earrings in that same way. Your face is your picture for life, and the accessories (hairstyle, earrings, etc.) are what frames it for the whole world to see. Earrings are that extra icing on the cake, and the special "giftwrap" trim that turns your face into a "special package."

A face is enhanced by the addition of an exciting color or the luminous shine reflected from precious metals like silver and gold.

Any old outfit is immediately updated with very little expense when pulled together with new and modern ear adornments.

By drawing attention to your face, you reflect your own personal image, style, and message in all situations: Casual, dressy, or professional.

Today's woman on the go knows that earrings are just as important with a warmup suit at the grocery store, as they are with a formal sequin gown at a carnival ball. The only difference is LIFESTYLE!

Eight

PICKING THE PERFECT PAIR...

Selecting just the right accessories, especially earrings, can be a difficult chore for many women. Sometimes you'll try on dozens of pairs without finding "just the right one," without ever realizing the true reason behind the confusion.

Often women limit themselves by being afraid to venture out to try something new, something larger than usual, or a new shape or color. Basically, that fear comes from the fact that the average woman does not know how earrings affect the overall appearance of the face, and accentuate the best features.

This guide book is created not only to help you determine your own face shape, but also to assist you in selecting the most flattering earrings for you. There are tips on why to wear, where to wear, and what to wear. You'll find instructions on how to completely re-do your current earring wardrobe, without having to throw away any of your old favorites. A simple alteration of earring backs, or the easy addition of a diskie or pad, will update items, and add years to their fashion life.

WHEN TO WEAR WHAT...

Most business situations call for earrings that are simple in style and design, not too casual, glitzy, or distracting with movement. They can range from the size of a dot up to a half dollar, and still be appropriate for most occupations. Basics, of course, are gold, silver, or pearls—definitely no fun plastics!

Plastic, wood, and leather designs are best worn for casual occasions, and selected to match and enhance the colors of your clothing. If you've had your colors analyzed professionally, you probably already know which tones look best with your skin. (Warm takes to gold, cool prefers silver.)

Women who look good in bright colors will look good in earrings of shiny metals, and women who look better in muted colors, should select ones with a duller or satin, antique finish that will not appear overpowering.

Hair color sometimes plays a role in picking that perfect color also. Gray, white, or silver haired ladies tend to especially glow in silver metals, while blondes favor gold. Red-heads and warm brown haired girls can usually choose bronze, copper, and wood that will highlight the texture and shade of their locks, but both gold and silver will be attractive on them also.

Rhinestones, jewels, beads, and crystal earrings will add a special glow that will flatter any face when chosen to match skin tones, hair shades, and wardrobe selection.

Ten

WHAT SIZE IS RIGHT???

The correct earring size is always a difficult decision to make. Very tiny dots do very little to enhance or show off facial features, but then sometimes long shoulder dusters or hanging dangles not only make a person look ridiculous, they also draw unwanted attention to sagging chins by visually pulling the face downward.

Don't listen to rumors, any woman can wear hoops, depending on the width and length of those hoops.

Try on different shapes and sizes in front of a mirror, and a friend! Let each help you decide what looks best. Women with large earlobes need at least a size to totally cover the bottom of the lobe. Women with tiny earlobes may be forced to wear pierced earrings, just to keep them on. The addition of earring backs and pads may solve this dilemma. (Note the chart below—for the different earring types and backs.)

In accessorizing it is wise to remember less is more. When wearing large or very eye catching earrings, do not overload with too many other accents. Sometimes just a simple scarf and a bracelet is more than enough to balance a silhouette. It is important that you select all accessories that flatter, that fit, and that make you look your very best.

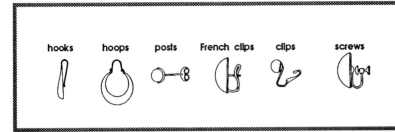

hooks   hoops   posts   French clips   clips   screws

Eleven

EARRINGS
AND THE SHAPE
OF YOUR FACE

One of the best reasons for wearing the right earrings is that they can actually alter the appearance of the face and head, particularly in terms of shape. By choosing the right earrings, the face can be made to look slimmer or wider, larger or smaller, whatever the intended goal. In addition, the ears and nose can be made to appear smaller by wearing larger sized earrings to create visual balance.

These ideas can be understood by learning how predominant lines—horizontal (—), vertical (|), curved (( ), and diagonal (/)—affect the apparent shape of the face. This can be achieved because the eye follows any predominant line or shape. (The idea of predominant lines and shapes are explained further in this booklet.)

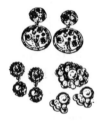 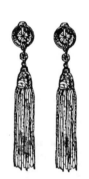 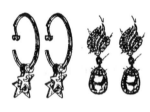

LINES
"PREDOMINANT LINES"

Understanding the concept of predominant lines and how they affect your face is the key to choosing the right earrings.

Remember the four types of lines you should be familiar with: Horizontal, vertical, diagonal, and curved. Since the eye follows the predominant or strongest line in an image, an earring with a certain line to it will have a given effect on the apparent shape of the face.

A predominant line can make your face and head appear longer and slimmer, or shorter and wider. Lines and shapes can also make the nose and ears seem smaller or larger. For example, balancing a large or protruding ear with a larger earring will make the ear appear smaller in comparison. At the same time, it may make the nose seem smaller.

Remember that the visual line may be formed by the actual structural shape of the earring, or it may be a line within the earring (such as a decorative design).

Examples:

Actual Shape

Decorative Line That Makes
The Earring Look Longer

Decorative Line That Makes
The Earring Look Shorter

FACE FACTS
DETERMINING YOUR FACE SHAPE

Method 1: Looking into a mirror, pull all of your hair away from your face with a headband or clips. While squinting one eye, trace on the mirror with soap or lipstick the general outline of your face. (See illustration.)

Method 2: Tie a brightly colored yarn (like the thick yarn for wrapping gifts) around your face and tie to hold it at the top of your head. (See illustration.) Be sure the yarn is along the sides of your face and just under the chin. With the yarn in place, take a close look at the shape of the face.

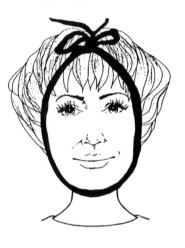

With either of these methods you should get a fairly general idea of the shape of your face. Be sure to take note of the wide and narrow points. Examine whether these points are at the forehead, cheekbones or chin line. As for the chin, look to see if it is narrow, rounded or squared.

FACE SHAPES
WHICH IS YOURS?

Even after you've used one of the two methods for determining your face shape, you may still be a little unsure of the particular shape of your face. That's only natural since most faces are not exactly one shape; that is, a face may not have every single characteristic of a particular shape. Your goal is simply to observe the face shape that most closely matches your own.

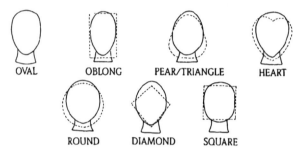

OVAL OBLONG PEAR/TRIANGLE HEART

ROUND DIAMOND SQUARE

TWO RULES TO REMEMBER

1. Although the general shape of the face is important, don't forget to consider these other factors: Your hairstyle, the length of your neck, the size of your ears, earlobes and nose. A special note about the neck: It may appear long or short, depending on whether the chin is small or recessed, full or double.

2. In trying to match the shape of your face with the shape of earrings, the most important rule to remember is: Do not repeat a pattern! Never use an earring shape that is the same as your face shape. By doing this, you would be emphasizing or exaggerating, rather than minimizing, the shape of your face.

Fifteen

OVAL SHAPE

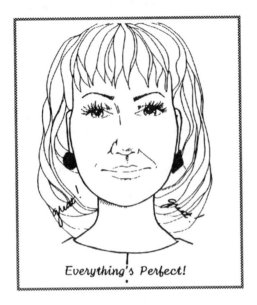

Everything's Perfect!

The oval-shaped face is the ideal face shape. It is usually two-thirds as wide as it is long. This face shape is slightly wider at the forehead, and the chin is only slightly narrowed.

In the oval-shaped face, the distance from the hairline to the eyebrow, from the eyebrow to the tip of the nose, and from the nose to the chin form nearly equal thirds. Note that the spacing of the eyes and the length of the nose can sometimes give the oval-shaped face a slightly different appearance.

The type of earring recommended: If the nose and ears are of average size, any style of earring may be worn.

SQUARE SHAPE

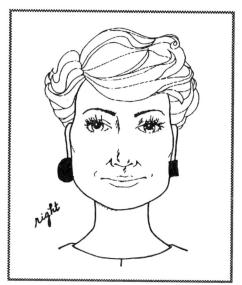

right

The square-shaped face is almost equal in length and width. The jaw may also appear squared, and with age, this squaring may become more pronounced.

Your Goal: To slim the face and give the jaw a less angular appearance.

How: Use earrings with vertical (I) and curved ( )) lines to make the face appear longer than it is wide. Avoid wearing earrings with an angular appearance.

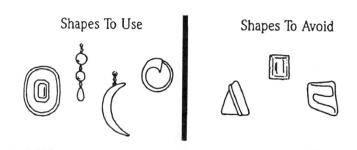

Shapes To Use   Shapes To Avoid

ROUND SHAPE

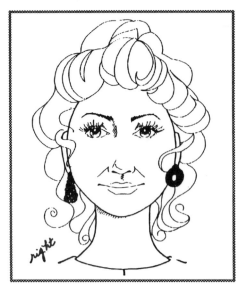

The round-shaped face is usually equal in roundness. Typically, the chin is not angular, but soft-looking. Quite often, although not always, women with this type of face also have relatively short necks.

Your Goal: To slim down the face and add angles to make it appear less rounded.

How: Choose earrings with vertical (I) lines and, when possible, those that are more angular in appearance. Avoid wearing earrings with curved ( ) lines since they will add roundness to the face.

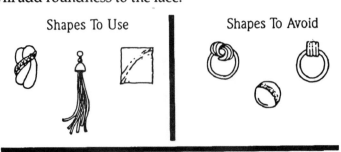

Shapes To Use   Shapes To Avoid

HEART SHAPE

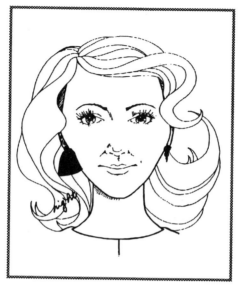

This type of face is generally wide at the top and narrow at the chin. The forehead may not necessarily be high, but it will usually be wider at the top and temple areas.

Your Goal: To widen and fill in the jaw line.

How: Select earrings that add both width and length. Triangles are especially good choices.

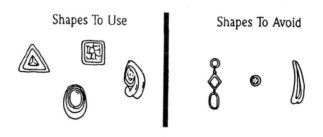

Shapes To Use   Shapes To Avoid

DIAMOND SHAPE

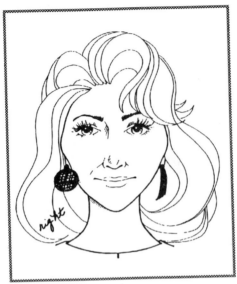

The diamond-shaped face is similar in appearance to the heart-shaped face with one difference. In the diamond-shaped face, the forehead is narrow, and the widest point is at the cheekbones.

Your Goal: To fill in and widen the jaw line and to give the face a less angular appearance.

How: Use earrings with softer or curved (( ) lines. Diagonal lines pointing outward are often recommended.

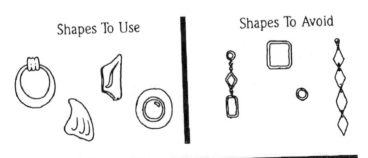

Shapes To Use

Shapes To Avoid

PEAR/TRIANGLE SHAPE

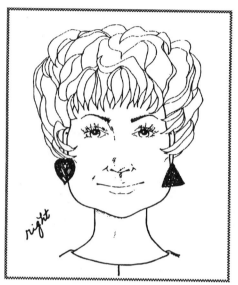

This type of face is full and round at the cheeks and chin, but becomes narrower at the forehead.

Your Goal: To slim down the cheeks, reducing the "cheeky" appearance of the face.

How: Choose earrings with vertical (I) lines. Avoid wearing round or wide earrings since they have a tendency to make the cheeks appear even fuller.

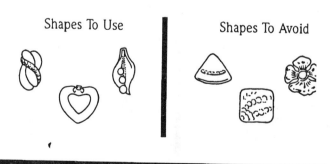

Shapes To Use   Shapes To Avoid

OBLONG SHAPE

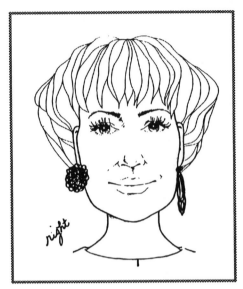

The oblong-shaped face is quite a bit longer than it is wide.

Your Goal: To shorten and widen the appearance of the face.

How: Select earrings with horizontal (—) lines and those in larger styles to fill in the extra length at the bottom of the face. Avoid choosing earrings with vertical (I) lines since they will make the face appear longer.

Shapes To Use   Shapes To Avoid

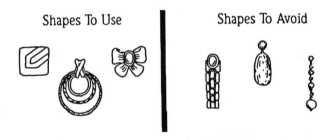

EARRING ADD-ONS
for EASY WEARING...

N ow that we've learned to pick the perfect pair, what happens when it's still not what we want? When I find just the right earring, it's usually pierced (and I only wear clip), or it is clip but it hangs off my ear or doesn't sit in the right place to flatter my face.

All problems can be easily corrected. To make an earring right, pull off the back (a pair of little pliers, a nailfile, or even a dull steak knife will do the trick), then use a strong adhesive to anchor it back in the right place. I prefer to use a glue gun with acrylic glue sticks, but a lot of people use E-2000 or E-6000, both glues are available at a local craft shop, variety store, or fabric center.

Remember you either remove the present pierce back and reuse it, if it is still in good condition, or replace it with a new one, pierced or clip, whichever fits your need.

A lot of pierced earrings tend to fall forward, not lying close to the earlobe. It is probably because the back clasp does not fit properly or it is too small to hold the weight of the earring. That's where diskies come in. Replace the regular pierced earring back (which is usually a small little gold squeeze-cap), with the round plastic circle, and see how much better your ear adornments stay in place.

Clip earrings are made for women who do not have pierced ears, or for those who wear heavy or large earrings. I personally just like the feel of a clip, but some complain they are uncomfortable or tend to fall off easily. To solve this, a slip-on ear pad will help secure the earring in place by adding that extra little cushioning. For comfortable wearing, the stick-on pads can also be used, but their main objective is to help the wearer who has a sensitivity to the metals of earrings. The stick-on pad will shield the skin from ever coming in contact with the actual earring, acting as a buffer to prevent any allergic reactions.

THE EXTRAS THAT MAKE EARRINGS EASY TO WEAR!

TRAVEL AND CARE OF EARRINGS

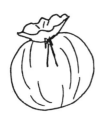

Since I travel so often, and because I pay quite a bit for my favorite earrings, it is very important to me that they are carefully packed during my travels. I have found the easiest way is to use one of the little bags that come in satin with a drawstring, and divided into individual pockets for earrings, necklaces, etc. They fit wonderfully in a suitcase and keep all valuables carefully separated.

At home, I like to see what I have to choose from, so I keep earrings out in clear view. There are several options, either using something like an earring organizer, which features not only holes for earrings but also end hooks for chains and a separate drawer for other goodies, or the TRIDANGLE which is a three sided stand- up display that will hold over 100 pairs of earrings—any style: Clip, pierced, studs, hooks, or posts fit into this slotted figure that stands 9" high.

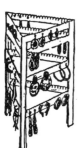

For the woman who has everything (as in lots of earrings), there is a hang-up bag that features about 40 see-through pockets, each with a zipper to keep earrings in place. This holder comes in handy for travel or can be hung anywhere for a clear view of your earring wardrobe.

Proper storage and care makes earring wearing a daily habit, as simple as brushing your teeth or washing your face. NEVER LEAVE HOME WITHOUT THEM.

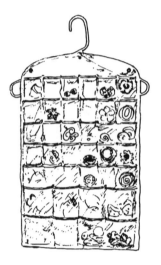

FRAMING THE FACE
A NOTE ABOUT GLASSES

At age twelve my first reaction to requiring prescription eyeglasses was one of horror and dread. I wanted to quit junior high and join a convent. Thank goodness, those days are long gone, and women no longer worry about the old wives tale, "Men won't make passes at girls who wear glasses."

Today's eyeglass wardrobes are considered accessories rather than necessities with many fashionable 90's ladies opting for clear glasses (make-believes) just to present a professional look. (Contact lens sales are down as it becomes in vogue to appear intelligent—I spent half of 1959 in tears for nothing!)

Here are a few basic rules in selecting frames that will flatter and frame your face:

✳ Let glasses compliment your skin tone and hair color, not your outfit. It's too expensive to try to color-coordinate your GLASSES to your wardrobe. Draw attention to your features—not fashions.

✳ Apply the rules of color analysis when selecting metal frames or trim—a warm tone complexion looks best in gold, while cool tones favor silver.

✳ Choose a shape which follows the natural curve of your brow line, with your eye centered in the lens. Glasses can balance your face and enhance or distract from features. Just like earrings, frames affect your appearance—they can widen, shorten, or lengthen your face visually. (Easier, cheaper, and less painful than plastic surgery any day!)

❋ Always remember to wear prescription shades or just regular sunglasses in the snow or sun to protect both your eyes and skin. That sensitive area just under the lower lash is the first to show signs of age. Prevent those little wrinkles from an early appearance, while enjoying the mysterious look of a "lady behind the lens." There's a certain glamour in wearing sunglasses. (Greta Garbo never left home without them!)

❋ If you only require reading glasses, please wear them with a certain flair. Your choices are so varied today, look for unique and unusual frames, and avoid a Ben Franklin impersonation. For fun, try some of those tiny ones sprinkled with glitzy stones. Also avoid letting them bounce around on a chain across your bodice. Remember, accessories draw attention. Unless you are trying to accent your bustline, I suggest reading glasses be put away in a case, or hung on one of those fashionable eyeglass hooks, worn as a pin.

❋ Although they are expensive, do try to have more than one pair of glasses. It is nice to be able to have a dressy and sporty choice when making a day-into-evening transition, and to avoid the boredom of the same old pair.

THIS IS A FASHION STATEMENT—FRAME THAT FACE!

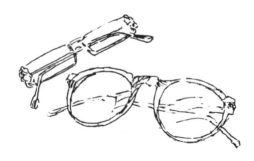

Twenty-Eight

THE NEW LOOK OF SCARVES

The easiest way to completely change a total look is by adding a brightly colored oblong at the waistline or a polka dot scarf at the neck. Scarves can take you from office to dinner in the same dress by creating a brand new image.

Color analysts suggest the use of scarves to shield unflattering shades away from the face. If you've just discovered you're a spring who should never wear black, don't throw away all your favorite black things. Just find scarves to compliment and coordinate. Throughout this section I'll show you how to use oblongs, scarves, shawls, and the little extra accessories such as bowmakers, sta-scarves, and hangerchiefs that'll make life easier.

A HANGERCHIEF is a large hanger that is available in a rainbow of colors at your local specialty shop or department store. It has 28 quarter-size holes to keep scarves, ties, and other accessory goodies hanging straight and in open view in your closet. No more drawers full of scarves, but nothing to wear. No excuse now for wrinkles, as this gadget keeps them all neat and ready to throw on at a moment's notice. (The hanger is also ideal for men's ties and belts, but don't let him use yours—buy two!)

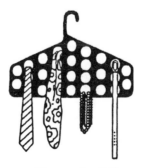

Twenty-Nine

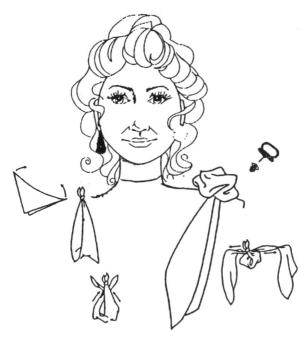

THE ROSE SCARF TRICK is definitely the most popular design in scarf tying today. Using a 36" square or larger, you can create your own rose garden without any shovel, dirt, or grass stained knees. I prefer to work with silk because it slides easier, but a polyester will achieve the same results. Fold the square into a triangle, and tie a loop at the top, leaving a tail of approximately 4". Holding over your hand, slide left end under knot and out the other side, hold, and then pull right end under knot, and out the other side. You will be holding a basket looking creation with two ends and the original loop you tied. Hold the two ends, shaking softly—it's in the wrist action—as the loop slides down the center. Give it a gentle pull, and slowly flip over and see your flower bloom. When you separate the tails, they become the leaves of the rose, and it is now ready to pin on a shoulder, a waistline as a belt, a decoration on a hat, and the perfect headband for a high fashion look. It is best held in place with a BETTEJON Sta-Scarf pin.

Thirty

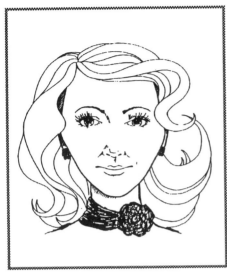

THE ROSE NECKLACE

For an oblong: place the scarf around your neck with both ends meeting down the front even. Loop together, and twist ends until they automatically begin to coil up. Continue to curl forming a circle rosette. Tuck the remaining small end into the center of the flower from underneath.

Using a square: Fold the two diagonal opposite points of a square in the middle to form an oblong. Circle around the neck and twist the ends until tight. Coil into a rosette design and tuck ends under.

THE NECKLINE FLOWER

Using a 36" square, folded into an oblong, place the scarf around the neck. with one end longer than the other. Tie a half-bow and fluff it out creating a flower-like puff. Adjust one side and drape remainder of the scarf down the front of the shoulder. Accent the center of the bloom with a pin, or use an old earring.

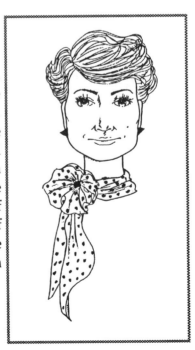

Thirty-One

THE SQUARE SCOUT

Nothing complicated about America's most popular scarf trick. Most people learned this basic as a child in Brownies or Girl Scouts. Fold any square into a triangle and drape the short point down the back, with ends running down front. The scarf should lay flat across the shoulders. Bring inside points together at the midway point between neck and scarf ends and make a square knot. (i.e. flip one end over the other, take upper end around and behind the other; pull through and tighten.)

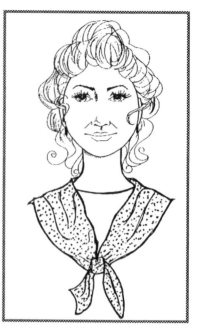

THE BUTTERFLY FAN

Using a folded square or an oblong, place the scarf around the neck and flip one end over the other so that the top piece is 5-9" long, the bottom should be much longer. Hand fold and accordian pleat the bottom part all the way up to the flip knot, then wrap the short end over the pleats and slip it through the loop to tighten. Fan out for a neat butterfly effect or turn to the side for a pleated bow look.

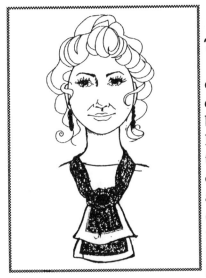

THE DOUBLE OVER

What's better than an oblong flip? A double flip, of course! Any 30" oblong can be beautiful. Also a 36" or longer square can be folded to acieve this hand-over design. Drape the scarf around the neck with ends even in the front. Flip the right end over left to form a half knot at the bustline level. Straighten the scarf ends so that the outer end is about 3" shorter than inner end. Hold the half knot and flip ends over your hand, and behind the knot. Adjust both ends, fan out fold and secure in place with a brooch or whimsical pin. (Even an extra earring will make a terrific and innovative decoration.)

THE NO-TIE SCARF

No work is required for this easy flip-over with an oblong scarf. Place the center of the long scarf around the neck in front and cross the ends behind the neck. Then drape to the front, let ends hang loose and a no-effort casual look has been achieved. To ·make a more cowl neck look, flip ends to back again and tie a tiny knot to hold in place. Hide the knot under the drape.

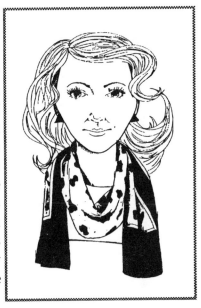

Thirty-Three

THE SCARF BLOUSE

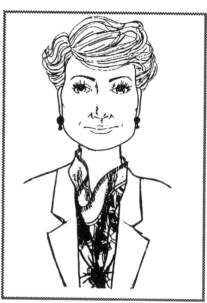

When traveling it is wonderful to use an extra scarf as a blouse for a change of looks. Simply take a square (the longer the better) and tie the ends around the neck, and the opposite ends around the waist, in the back. Blouse out the fabric for a softer look, put on a jacket, and no one will ever suspect it's not a blouse.

THE DOUBLE SCOUT or COWL

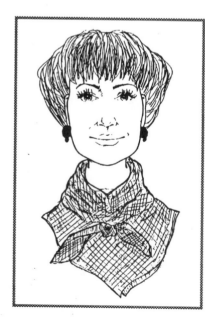

This is a reverse of the Square Scout. Fold a scarf into a triangle, but this time drape the short end down the front and two longer ends over the shoulder to the back. Instead of tying, cross over to the front, then tie a single small knot at the throat. For a softer ascot look, drape the fabric nearest the chin over the knot.

WEAR and CARE
of SCARVES

When you purchase a new scarf, be sure to check the care label as soon as you return home. Then IMMEDIATELY, cut or tear it out. This is a care label, not some status name-tag. There is nothing worse than a beautifully tied scarf with a name tag reading 100% silk. (Yes, there is something worse; it could be polyester!) Don't wear these tags as accessories!

I suggest that you take an index card and write a description of the scarf, and then attach the label for safe keeping. Then you can refer to it if the scarf becomes soiled. (Again, I REPEAT—rip off the label. This is not a mattress. The police are not coming to issue you a citation!)

Pure-silk scarves usually require dry cleaning, although some can be washed gently in cool water. I would possibly do this with a solid color, hand washing in a very mild detergent. Otherwise, I'd feel safer paying the dry cleaning bill. Most silks are expensive and should be treated as a prize possession.

Polyester or acrylic scarves may be hand washed or even possibly machine washed in cool water, on gentle cycle. Avoid squeezing or wringing scarves. Rinse thoroughly; excess water may be removed by rolling flat in a towel. Drip dry, and iron on a low setting.

In planning your scarf wardrobe, take note: silk scarves are thin, while polyester ones are much thicker. A short neck requires a silk, whereas you lucky long neck girls can opt for the savings of polyester's lower price tags.

PIN-UPS

Pins are used to reflect personality, express a mood, and define a look. Picking the perfect pin is the final touch to completing an outfit.

Most pins are worn either in the center or off to the left of a lapel or at mid shoulder. There is nothing more lovely than an antique cameo on the high collar of a romantic lace collared blouse, or a decorative shoulder pin, but if placed just like a convention name badge, these may be considered stylish, but... they're also d-u-l-l! I like fun, fashion, and fabulous!

It is said that 94% of all American women have medium or sloping shoulders. This figure fault makes it imperative that some type of shoulder pad be worn to give a taller, trimmer, more balanced silhouette. If the accent pin is placed on the outer edge of the shoulder, it will give the illusion of more width. The higher the pin is placed, the taller the wearer will appear, as eyes will be drawn upward. (Use those gorgeous pins to offset a not-so-attractive hipline!)

In my video, THE ACCESSORY ADVANTAGE: TACKY TO TERRIFIC, I am seen wearing a large black and white geometric shape high on my shoulder. This creation by Deborah Holbrook is a delightful design of beads, fabric, chain, and even bits of silver cord, which makes it a whimsical finishing touch to my otherwise very classic herringbone blazer. Pins such as this can turn a uniform or a basic plain outfit into a fashion statement.

A different approach to accents is clustering. The more the better, is a good motto when placing scatter pins all over an outfit. A blazer pocket can be personalized with tiny hearts or a small zoo of miniature animals. A masculine tie is a super menswear look, but is immediately made feminine with the addition of several small stickpins or tie tacs.

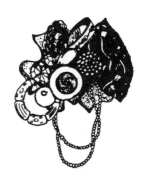

The CLIP-IT is a take-off of the old sweater guard from years ago, but it can be worn to nip in the waist of a garment, draw interest to a five-pocket jean, and even decorate a neckline as it's chain spans across a tie from collar tip to collar tip.

Holding a scarf in place with a pin is old news, but it can be new again if it is the right pin. A large gold safety pin trimmed in stones is fantastic on a heavy wool wrap. A delicate silver floral design is ideal to create a soft drape in a silk ascot. Use pins to highlight colors, textures, and designs of scarves.

Don't forget the element of surprise in your pin wardrobe. I am well-known for my spider collection (over twenty little creatures in gold, silver, and stones). I use these pins to make a great impression coming and going, so I frequently wear one of the little bugs on the upper left back of my shoulder (not quite on top—more like crawling upward!). It's an unusual touch, and creates fashion fun attention. Pins can also be used on the cuff or sleeve edge for different highlights.

Let's not forget the hands! Fashion on the fingertips doesn't have to mean rings. Why not pin an antique brooch on your glove? Use one as an added accessory to your evening bag. A rhinestone glitter item will take a plain fabric bag from day into evening with that needed touch of glamour!

Pins don't always have to be pins either. I sometimes use pierced earrings and simply add a little rubber back to secure it in place. Look through that jewelry collection.

Thirty-Seven

There's probably a total new look just waiting to be discovered and used!

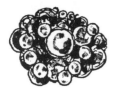 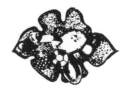 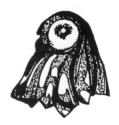

PUSH-UP to PERFECTION!

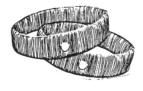

Several years ago I came across a simple pair of push-ups which actually changed my life. No, not the kind you do on the floor, a la Jack Palance at the Academy Awards; the kind you wear. When I first laid eyes on that pair of gold sleevebands, I knew my future was set as an image consultant. I spent the next few years singing their praises to everyone who would listen. This innovative metal elastic cuff was a discovery which has delighted women nationwide.

How can a little band make such a big difference? Just slip one over your garment sleeve and push up. You'll have a fashionably secure look (and feeling)—no more creeping down or dropping sleeves. You 'll no longer have to roll a cuff, exposing an ugly lining; no more cutting off the circulation with rubber bands. (Rubber bands will also tear and ruin your fabric or pop off at any time.) Just ask Paula Zahn!

One day I was watching the CBS Morning Show when Harry Smith let out a little "ouch!" Paul Zahn then giggled, and revealed to her millions of viewers that she had been holding up her sleeves with rubber bands and one had popped, hitting Harry. I was amazed that this million dollar anchor woman was not aware of this inexpensive accessory necessity, so I immediately overnighted her a pair by UPS. Soon I received a handwritten note on CBS stationary which I have framed and hanging in my office. It reads, "Thank you for solving my problems! Sincerely, Paula."

Besides saving face in a funny situation, these bands do make you look taller, trimmer, and better dressed. There is an old saying, *"Never wear anything you gotta fiddle with."* For non-Southerners that means, *"Don't play with your clothes."* If you have to constantly touch or tug on something, take it off. Sleevebands eliminate that horrible habit of pushing up that falling sleeve. They are ideal for casual looks and career wear. The accent away from the hipline when fabric is pushed up, gives the illusion of a slimmer body.

Most companies offer bands in many colors, ranging from gold, silver, or black, to even the fashion hues like royal, pink or purple. I've seen them designed with jewels, buttons, bows, and bells, BUT... THEY SHOULD NOT SHOW! If someone can see them, you have them on wrong, so what difference does it make about what color they are?

Color doesn't matter, but you do need several pair. (I loved it when Rue McClanahan purchased a dozen. I always wondered if they were all for her or if she shared them with The Golden Girls.) The bands are so attractive, they have many uses: They can double as bracelets when necessary or serve as ankle bands for a quick alteration of slacks that are too long. I've seen women who have used them to add a feminine puff sleeve when wearing a mans oversize tee-shirt, and once, I must confess, my husband had to wear them under his suit jacket when I forgot to have the sleeves of his new dress shirt hemmed in time for a special occasion. It worked!

People constantly share with me other wonderful ways to use these little treasures. For bikers, it keeps their

Forty

pants leg from being caught in the spokes. For golfers, the wet grass and morning dew will not stain trousers. Find your own new and unusual way to make use of a pair.

Sleevebands, Sleeve Garters, Armbands, Push-Ups..., no matter what you call these simple little circles, they are a miracle with a multitude of uses in your wardrobe.

BELTED BODIES

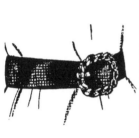

Although the larger woman needs to pay close attention to her belt selection, there is a style on the market available to everyone. Perhaps the easiest to wear is a stretch belt either in elastic or fishscale metal because it will contour to the body, giving proper room for fit and comfort. This one-size-fits-most style is always my favorite because this belt will caress a body—not strangle it!

Any waistline looks better with some definition. A contrast color will call attention to a tiny waist, while a self-fabric one is best to camouflage. A tight belt on a small waist will make large hips look even more out-of-proportion. I prefer to wear my belt a bit looser, angled down off to one side for a lowered waistline effect. This also will visually lengthen a short waist.

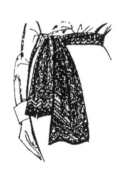

Another illusion to appear longer waisted is to wear a belt the same color as your top. (To lengthen legs, do the opposite, matching the waist accent to the pant or skirt.)

OMEGA, one of America's top manufacturers of moderate-to-better priced belts, suggests the following when looking for the right belt:

❋ Stretch belts are generally made of poly-elastic which provides give and size-memory. This type works with almost all body types. Traditionally the most comfortable and important width is 2 inches, although 1 to 1-

1/4-inch versions are great with pant or shorts looks. The younger woman or those who are tall and thin can also enjoy a more dramatic 3-inch belt design in this style.

✳ Chain belts are constructed from a variety of different metals and are usually gold or nickel plated. Chain styles allow great flexibility of size because they can be worn high on the waist or slung low around the hips to flatter individual figures. Consider chain 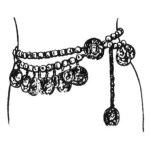 belts as jewelry, always trying to coordinate with earrings or necklaces. Chains can be worn with dresses, suits, and for a more tailored look—pants. For the model figure, chain belts are the ideal accent with a bodysuit, stirrup pants, or lycra dressing.

✳ The pant belt gets its name because of its ability to fit through trouser (or skirt) loops. The typical width is 1 to 1-1/3 inches. This is considered the basic belt of every woman's ward-robe. This is the accessory needed in a variety of colors, textures, and buckle treatments. Pant belts exist in career, casual, and dressy evening looks and are usually sized to the waist. A correct fit is determined by buckling the belt in the center hole. (No tab left over? You need a larger size. Excess flap? Go down a size!)

✳ The suit belt is a more "career" look, and is usually 1-1/2 to 2 inches in width. Suit belts are made of smooth, textured, suede, or patent materials. Buckles can be either self-covered (the most conservative) or bold in dramatic gold or silver.

✳ A cummerbund or wrap-belt is a silhouette that is dramatic and bold. Often they are from 2 to 4 inches in width and made of soft fabric or leather, or a mixture of cording, metal, wood, or jewel details. Traditionally this type either buckles, snaps, or works with a velcro closure.

When a jacket is worn, only a small section of any belt is visible. Even a thick waist will have the illusion of slimness when only four inches are showing! Don't give up belted bodies, just learn to coverup the negatives and accentuate the positives.

HANDBAG
HAPPINESS

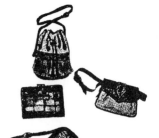

No segment on fashion or accessories would be complete without mention of that MOST IMPORTANT addition—the handbag. Have you ever noticed that earrings can be forgotten, belts may fall by the wayside, legs often remain bared, but seldom will a woman leave her home without a handbag?

In my grandmother's day they were called "pocketbooks"—then the word "purse" came into vogue. Now to keep pace with the changing fashion lingo, it is a "handbag."

This seemingly simple accessory is perhaps the most difficult purchase for most shoppers. There are so many factors to consider: Size, color, price, texture, the overall total look. It's important to buy the best you can afford, since most women HATE to change bags. Still, don't try to fool yourself into thinking, there is one bag for everything—THERE IS NO SUCH THING!

A bare wardrobe necessity would be two bags—a good leather for career and dress, and a tote or straw basket style for casual everyday use. Shoes and bags no longer have to match, as long as they coordinate and blend. Fabric, design, and shape will determine which bag is best for your lifestyle needs.

For some odd reason, most women think bags come with labels that read: "Fill 'til full." Are you guilty of this handbag overload? (Don't start with the excuses. I don't want to hear about your five block morning walk in high heels or how you carry your lunch to the office.) Not only is this oversized sack T-A-C-K-Y, it could be seriously harmful to your health. It's uncomfortable, and physically impossible to lug around half a house, when a compact, wallet, car keys, and checkbook would be sufficient. (Please refer to the hosiery chapter to see my advice about the other item to carry in your handbag.)

This is only a handbag; it can't work miracles. If you're headed to the office—GET A BRIEFCASE! If you have a baby—USE A DIAPER BAG! If you are running away from home—CARRY A SUITCASE!

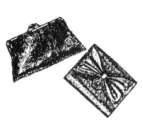

Most image consultants concur, the ideal figure flattering bag is no more than 10" high, no longer than 12", or thicker than 3". (That's bigger than you think, I promise!) Try on handbags when shopping, just as you would garments. Look into the three way mirror. See how you look coming and going. Consider your total body silhouette when selecting this important accessory. Unlike that blouse that you may wear once every two weeks, a handbag is with you almost every day.

P.S. In my seminars and workshops, I always enjoy selecting handbags from the audience participants. I am constantly amazed at what some women will carry around all day, and equally surprised at how they manage it. A word to the 'wide:' If your hips are large, don't allow a bag to bump up against them. This only draws additional attention to your widest area. Have the shoulder straps shortened so the bag will be at the center of your waistline, your smaller and more flattering spot.

If your bust line is more than ample, don't dare tuck that clutch under your arm—it looks like you have three across. (Get the picture? Everyone else does, and it ain't pretty!)

HAPPY HEMLINES
and LEGS TO MATCH

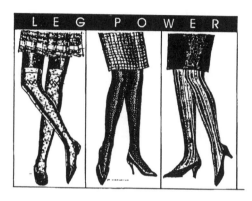

Skirts are up; skirts are down; you never know what's in style when. Since designers never seem to be able to agree on the proper length, may I suggest you find the most flattering for your body—and stick with it! That's usually about one to two inches below the knee cap where the leg begins to curve. Forget what CALVIN says, and take a long hard look at yourself in a full length mirror. Are those knees ready to meet the public? (Mine aren't!) Are you willing to expose yourself for fashion's whim? If you like what you see, and have the confidence to bare thighs, GO FOR IT! If not, never fear. Leggings, thigh huggers, knee socks, pantyhose, and other exciting leg accents will always be trendy.

I've discovered that illusions can be created with design patterns and textures of hose. A short woman or one with large calves looks better in hose and shoes of the same color. If the hosiery, the shoes, and the hemline all match, the look will be even taller and thinner. It's the break in the color tone that tends to chop us into sections, causing a short, dumpy effect.

This will always occur if hose are darker than your shoes. In other words, white hose with black shoes are fine, but black hose with white shoes are a definite no-no! (Think of all those Easter Sundays when some lady wore her new sailor dress with navy hose and white shoes. Didn't she look like she cruised in on two boats?)

When selecting hosiery, I follow the three "C" words in looking for cover-up, camouflage, and control top. There are some brands of pantyhose which can actually give the appearance of a five pound weight lost. (I prefer basic black or bit-of-black or barely black with re-enforced heel and toe, plus girdle top!) The sandalfoot hose are a necessity for shoes with the toe out, but how often do you wear sandals? Almost all of us are used to wearing a closed in pump, but still purchase sandalfoot hose without thinking. Remember re-enforced toe hose will last up to five times longer than sheer toe. (Follow that one tip, and you've already saved double the cost of this book in less than one month's hosiery bills!)

My personal hosiery law (I'm trying to get it passed in the Senate, but no luck so far), requires women to buy THREE pair at one time. A well-dressed woman is never fashionably secure without ONE pair on her body, ONE pair in her handbag, and ONE pair in her desk drawer or glove compartment of the car. Never spoil a special event in your life just because there's a runner up your leg. Make a quick change, and come back smiling!

There are many old wive's tales about the longevity of hosiery. It is said that they will wear longer if first put in the freezer, then defrosted and dried. (I tried it, I wore them four times—so who knows?) Washing hose in white vinegar is another suggestion which I tried. As the day wore on in our south Louisiana heat, I began to have the faint aroma of a dinner salad. So much for that idea!

Several years ago I did learn something from my teenage daughter about putting on stockings. I have long nails and was constantly snagging or even putting my entire finger through the sheers, until I saw her put on hers. She keeps a pair of white cotton gloves in her hosiery drawer and wears them each time she slips into her pantyhose. What a practical and sensible idea! No wonder she never seemed to wear out as many as I did. (Personally, I thought maybe the petite sizes lasted longer than the queen-size until I discovered the glove routine!)

The rules of hosiery have changed very little from my mother's generation to that of my daughter. Mother still claims (and she's backed up by MISS MANNERS) that it's "No white shoes 'til Memorial Day, and they must be packed away on Labor Day." This is an old strict rule of dress, especially in the South, but most folks have been lenient enough to begin at Easter, and then put into storage on Labor Day—(It's NOT just a Southern thing!)

Bare legs come under the same ruling, being acceptable from Memorial Day until Labor Day, but never in a professional wardrobe. A career woman should dress properly at all times; hosiery is a must, no matter what the temperature. Bare legs are also not acceptable in church (but that's just a personal opinion, and something my mother probably instilled in me years ago.)

Black hosiery (my favorite) was once considered too dark and heavy for summer time wear, but it's now fine all year round. For the cooler months, you may want to wear an opaque or thicker legging, but in summer black sheers are perfect to make legs appear slimmer.

Now white pantyhose, that's a pet peeve of mine! I figure they are for two people: nurses and twelve-year olds. Let 'em have them, and you select yours in shades called pearl, alabaster, creme. I promise these will give you the white look you are trying to achieve without the glare of the true white. Remember skin tones, when blended with sheer colors, will always appear a different shade. Trust me—no white!

Hemline borders on skirts have to be considered an

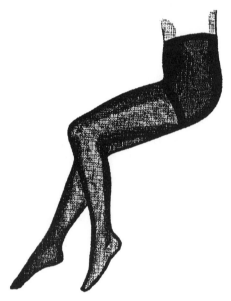

accessory item because they draw attention to the leg. Do you have great gams? Then spotlight them. If not, forget the bordering. Another leg look accessory is the ankle bracelet. (Unless you're going to a beach party and this is your wild and crazy fun look, forget it! That's another of those items that belong to teenagers, and do not age well!)

SECTION II

FUN

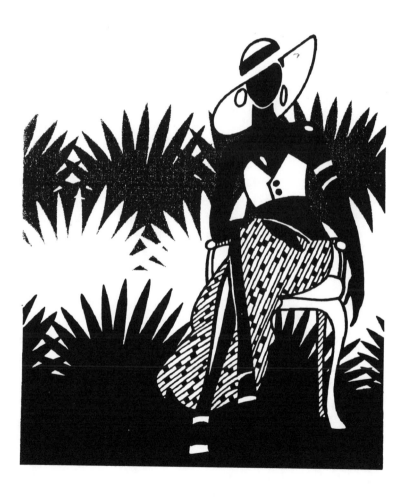

PROFESSIONAL
POLISH

Tips for Career Dressing

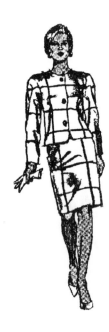

Recent surveys showed that two out of every three women in America, under age 55, are now employed full or part-time outside the home. As these statistics rise, more and more women are also entering a new world of fashion where the rules of dress are very different from their everyday leisure lifestyle. Many are finding themselves totally unprepared for professional dress. Those who can afford it are seeking the assistance of image consultants and personal shoppers to select their career clothing. Others are spending hours on end, searching for just the right thing for their daily uniform.

No longer are women a slave to the 1970's theory of DRESS FOR SUCCESS. Those navy blue IBM suits and men look-a-likes in pin-stripe or charcoal are a thing of the past. Even the most conservative corporate employee is now seen in softdressing (a silky skirt and blouse, topped with an unconstructed blazer.)

My friend, Gail Florin, founder of The Ideal Silhouette system of body analysis and author of the book of the same name, offered these suggestions for the nineties working woman:

Fifty-Two

(1) Do wear a watch. Not only is this a nice piece of jewelry, a professional needs to know what time it is. Punctuality is a must, as it shows a regard for others. Time is today's most valuable commodity. Use it wisely.

(2) Do not wear perfume. Many tend to disagree with this statement, but very few women understand what the term "lightly" means, so it is best to say NO perfume. Heavy perfume odors tend to give off sexual messages and can be considered offensive by both men and women. Don't risk losing a valuable account over a dab of Chanel #5; save it for a romantic evening.

(3) Don't wear distracting jewelry. If it shines, dangles, or jangles, leave it at home until after work hours. A business meeting does not need to be interrupted by a musical tune played as you walk across the room. Limit those bracelets to ONE silent cuff.

(4) Do keep nails well manicured, tapered medium length. Short, bitten nails are not only unattractive, they reveal a lack of self confidence and discipline. Long nails will interfere with your work, and appear unprofessional. Light colored polish is accepted, but steer clear of brights or frosted tones.

(5) A career shoe is no higher than 2 and 1/2 inches. It has a closed-in heel and toe. These are comfortable, fashionable, and flattering to the leg. Do check heels, keep repaired and clean. A sheet of "Bounce" or "Clingfree" fabric softener is an instant shoe polisher. Keep one handy in your briefcase or desk drawer.

(6) Do always keep an extra pair of nylons in your handbag, glove compartment, or desk drawer. Do not wear colored nylons or seamed and textured hosiery for business.

(7) Always carry a neat handbag or briefcase, but never both. A small clutch can hold makeup and wallet, and fit easily inside a briefcase. It is very awkward to shake hands holding both a briefcase and a handbag. When on non-business errands or going to lunch, use the clutch, leaving the briefcase in your office or car.

(8) Do wear a jacket or blazer on the job. It carries its own authority, making you well-dressed, and giving you a more secure fashion feeling of being "in charge" and "in style." (I repeat, you do not have to copy a man's mode of dress. Your jacket can be floral, solid, checked, whatever fits your mood and flair.)

(9) Pants are not generally acceptable in most offices and work places.If they are necessary for your occupation, the slacks should be well-tailored and softly pleated, never the least bit tight. Be careful to select the proper shoes and heel height for slacks.

(10) Don't select career garments that are sleeveless, wrapped, or revealing. Avoid neon colors and tight-fitting garments. Draw attention to your work, not your body.

(11) A perfect skirt length for career is the classic length: 2" inches below the knee cap. Skirts can be longer, but should not be much shorter. A professional should never ever expose her knee caps. Save those minis and walk shorts for after hours fun and leisure.

(12) For non-business occasions, do not wear your nine-to-five working wardrobe. You dress so much for career that the few times you can socialize, wear a dress or soft pants outfit. If your clothing budget forces you to mix/match skirts and blazers, do so, but try not to appear to be working during your off-hours activities. You will give the impression that you are networking and/or collecting business cards, rather than enjoying the company of others.

(13) Pay attention to the little things. Use a lint brush. Check for loose and missing buttons. Clean and air clothing after each wearing. (Any time you enter a building where people smoke, your clothing will automatically absorb these odors. If you then hang them in your closet, the odor will spread to your entire wardrobe.)

(14) "DRESS FOR THE JOB YOU WANT, NOT THE JOB YOU HAVE." You never know who's going to walk into your office or see you in an elevator. It may be the same person you see days later across the interview table. Dress prepared daily for that big break; you never know when it'll happen. Be ready!

(15) Remember those you love and live with. Don't make Saturday and Sunday a day to throw fashion to the winds. Why not look nice for those who care about you? Twenty years from now, the job may be gone and those people won't even remember your name, but the loved ones will cherish every memory of their weekends with you. Make the extra effort to fix your hair, put on makeup, and greet the weekend with the same care and concern you put into each work day!

(These suggestions are career DO'S & DON'TS for women in the professional world of banking, insurance, finance, legal affairs, engineering, stock market, etc. If you are a school teacher, a nurse, fashion sales clerk or other specialized field, a different set of dress code rules apply to your particular position. But, remember: *Being appropriately dressed is always acceptable, and never goes out of style.*)

A BASIC WARDROBE WITHOUT A BANK LOAN

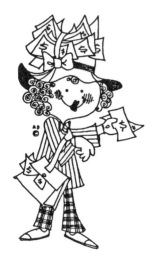

It is no laughing matter that today's shop-til-ya-drop generation of young women have now grown up to find they have "nothing to wear." Every morning in front of closets all across America, the cries are heard as career women push and pull hangers in desperation. They throw garments on the floor in a mad rush to find the perfect outfit for today's important job interview or this afternoon's special meeting. A recent magazine reported that the average working women spends about $150 a month on her career wardrobe, which is quite a hefty investment, considering her salary is estimated to average less than $18,000 annually.

Putting together a versatile, affordable, workable wardrobe is not as difficult as it may seem if a shopper follows a few basic fashion rules and consumer guidelines. Let's start with these suggestions.

Begin by cleaning your closets—all of them! Set aside a Saturday and start by completely emptying the contents onto the bed or the floor. Divide the clothing into category stacks. Anything that hasn't been worn in the last twelve months should be discarded at once—you certainly haven't missed it lately, have you? Next, get rid of anything that doesn't fit. Don't use that old diet-next-week excuse with me. You're not only setting yourself up for disappointment, you're cluttering up your closet space with daydreams. Get real; kiss the skinny stuff goodby. (Should you ever become that skinny again, you're going to buy all NEW clothes anyway, aren't ya?)

See—I've been there before—I know you!

Anything that needs cleaning, repairing, or altering should be delivered to the professional. Take it out to the car NOW so you won't forget!

If you have extra closets, put any out-of-season clothing out-of-sight. The idea here is to save time in the morning, not review a fashion catalogue of your wardrobe. Divide remaining items into categories such as tops, bottoms, jackets, dresses, jeans. Arrange them by color co-ordination for easy mix-match access.

This is the best time to determine if you have a good color basis forming in your clothing selections. (Ever look in your closet and realize EVERYTHING is purple, or a shade of?) By using two base colors with three of your most flattering fashion colors, you can build a complete look that will all work back together. You may want to use a small notebook to list items by type and color. (Don't feel stupid; all movie stars, rock stars, even Hillary Clinton, have clothing consultants who did this for them.)

Example: Blouse-red, slacks-blue; this is for your shopping references. (Again don't feel odd going into the store with a list. This is a time and mind saver. Your energy needs to be used for more important things!!) Look for gaps in your needs, and fill them. Consider both lifestyle and budget to determine shopping priorities as IMMEDIATE (you can not exist another day without), and FUTURE (would be nice to have).

Fifty-Seven

Most of us have a favorite item (mine is a fabulous b/w checked blazer) around which to build our wardrobe story and base. This garment should be of good quality, enduring style, and will probably be the most expensive item you purchase. Afterall, it is the center of your clothing investment portfolio. Requirements should include that it be well-constructed, easy-to-care for, durable, flattering, and versatile enough to mix-match with numerous colors. (If you've had your colors professionally analyzed, this will be a snap!)

When leaving home on this shopping expedition, take along both the favorite item (base piece) and the list you made during the closet cleaning. It's important to see how new items will blend with this wardrobe basic. Try it on with skirts, and slacks to make sure the lines blend, colors co-ordinate, and textures are compatible. It is unwise to buy odd pieces without at least one matching mate. Easy interchanging of garments will save closet space, shopping time, and most important—dollars. Don't get caught up in a "to-die-for mood" and purchase something that doesn't fit into your plan! (The object is to save time and money, freeing up funds for more fun!)

Before buying, check the care labels on all new purchases. A $49.99 blazer is certainly not a good buy if it will be at the dry cleaners more than in your closet or on your body. With the price of gasoline these days, even the trip to the laundry can be costly. Pay very close attention to fabrics and care labels in everthing. There is a real difference between washable silk and 100% silk.

Select accessories when you're buying your clothing. Belts, scarves, and jewelry can be the extenders for a sparse wardrobe budget. Get several different looks from dressy to casual, from preppie to ethnic, simply by accessorizing. Experiment with metals to discover if you're better in gold or silver for your personal choice. (Again a color analyst could answer this!) Dare to be different with accessorizing trends, but not outrageous. A working women's wardrobe should draw pleasing looks, not stares!

Here are the bare necessities I'd list for today's wardrobe:

- ✣ Two belts (one leather, one chain)
- ✣ Four scraves (One oblong, two square, one oversize)
- ✣ One strand of pearls
- ✣ One choker (gold or silver)
- ✣ Four pairs of earrings
- ✣ A lapel pin
- ✣ Two bracelets (perhaps one metal and one wood)

It is vital that two handbags be used—one casual, maybe a duffle or a tote, and one good leather classic bag. Don't scrimp on prices here; get the best you can afford. If possible, a wardrobe needs two watches: one with a leather band for casual play, and a better small gold or silver style for work and dress.

A baker's dozen of garments could be mix-matched into twenty-eight different looks if purchases are properly color co-ordinated. You'll need at least two dresses, hopefully one could be a two-piece style, useful for versatility with other pieces in your closet. I recommend two jackets—one in a solid basic such as navy, camel, or black, perhaps the other in a tweed or soft small check pattern. With these, you'll need two skirts, again a solid and maybe a small print, one pair of dress trousers in a basic color, and one pair of casual jeans or pants. To round out your clothing agenda you should have five tops—three blouse/shirt styles, and two knits or sweaters, depending on the season, or your local climate.

The possibilities are endless for coordinating each piece and creating a new and different look every day by the addition of a scarf or changing of a top. By having fewer garments to wade through each morning, you'll find your time is better spent making yourself as attractive and well-dressed as possible. You may find that by laying out your daily selections the night before, you'll be able to enjoy an extra special minute of beauty rest that'll add to your appearance as a well-groomed professional woman or happy homemaker!!

THE SOMETHING
MORE WOMAN

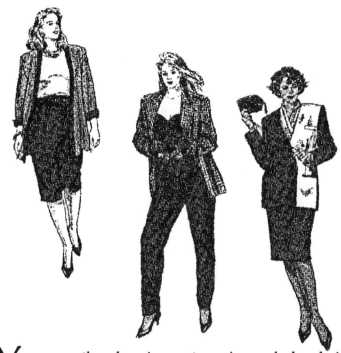

Years ago the plus size customer's wardrobe choices were limited to baggy shirtwaist shifts, oversized dolman sleeve tunics, and ill-fitting elastic waist pants, all available in dark colors or basic black!

Thank goodness, the dark ages are over as designers and manufacturers have begun to realize BIG CAN BE BEAUTIFUL, and PRETTY DOES NOT HAVE TO MEAN PETITE. It also helped that a recent survey showed that one-third of all the women in America wore a size 14 or larger. One in six women are a size 22 or more.

As one of those special size ladies, I felt like yelling, "Hip! Hip! (no pun intended) Hooray!" We're finally being acknowledged and recognized as a majority group in today's fashion world. Still, with over one-third of all women being classified as "something more," it remains a fact that 70 percent of all ladies apparel is designed and manufactured in size 12 or smaller.

The past chapters on accessorizing have been ideal to help the fuller-figure woman (like me) enhance the figure by maximizing the best features. Accessories accentuate the positives and minimize the negatives through the combination of proper design, shape, texture, and color.

Even if you feel that black dress is still the most slenderizing thing in your closet, let the accessories be the necessity that adds zest and life to an otherwise dull and boring outfit. A large pair of earrings, a long rope necklace, or a colorful oblong scarf can make the difference between appearing "fat and frumpy" or "tall and terrific!" (I know which one I'd choose.)

Follow along with me as I list tips especially for that one in three women who needs to know, BEAUTIFUL COMES IN ALL SIZES. Let's begin by reciting my favorite 'Bible' verse (from the book of *Chanel*!), "GOD MAKES— BUT APPAREL SHAPES." Don't you just love the sound of that? Take a long hard look at what God has given you, accept it with love, and begin to accent and show off your best attributes!

The key element to be considered by the SOMETHING MORE shopper (doesn't that sound so much nicer than PLUS SIZE?) is that vertical lines slim. Therefore, when selecting a new wardrobe, search for the up and down slender looks that will add height and drop pounds, visually. Be certain that any stripe garments fit without pulling or distorting the lines.

Solid separates with contrasting color tops and bottoms will create a broken line, thus cutting your silhouette in half. Wear narrow stripes; wide awning stripes up and down are just as unflattering as a horizonal line.

Long, fitted or slightly unconstructed jackets in a fingertip length will look nice, as will fitted sheaths and shifts. Long over lean adds height and creates optical illusions. Narrow bodice tucks and vertical pleats add a pleasing look; so does princess seaming and center front seams. Add spark to a simple shirtwaist by adding new button covers or rows of contrasting buttons for trim. If changing colors in tops and bottoms, keep light and bright on top nearer your face, and darker on bottom.

The most slimming skirt style for most size 16 ladies or larger is usually an A-line, which is more comfortable with an elastic waist. (Be sure to cover this with an attractive not-too-wide belt.) Personally, I've found I can wear a slim, straight skirt with a blazer, as long as the hipline is not too tight. Usually a good alteration person can insure that the waistband is taken in to fit, but why not ask them to also taper the bottom of the skirt? Beginning a couple of inches below the widest part of the thigh, taper in to a trimmer hemline. Two or three inches off that skirt width at the hem will work wonders in achieving the slim look you want. You can also wear a long, lean top in a relaxed silhouette (a cardigan, tee, tunic) over a softly pleated or flared skirt.

The less fuss and fabric on the fullness of your body, the better you look. Therefore, the best pocket is NO pocket, but the second choice to flatter is a hidden pocket, followed by a diagonal. Again ask that alteration expert to remove or simply sew-up pockets that can cause unsightly bulges of fabric on the side of your hip. It's a good way to keep you from sticking your hands in your pockets or worse yet, loading them down with keys, coins, or anything else that will make you appear larger than you actually are. At all costs, avoid a rounded curved pocket which will add inches and pounds to its location.

Long jackets are perfect for covering a multitude of sins, IF it is the right jacket for your body shape. Single-breasted designs fit almost every "body," but it takes extra height to carry off the two-button style of the double-breasted look.) Again, you don't need the extra fabric and bulk.) A cardigan is ideal because it seems to be the most slimming. It's collarless design can minimize a full bust, trim a full hipline, cover broad shoulders, and lengthen a short neck. (Sounds like a miracle, doesn't it?) Try one on today, and pick a bright alive color. Leave that dull black for someone in mourning!)

Straight leg or stove pipe pants will work best for the larger figure, but no cuffs are allowed. This will chop off your body at the ankles, as do contrast socks or hosiery between the hemline and shoes. Stirrup pants which have been so popular recently can be a good style, IF they are not worn too tight. The "v" effect of a long top over slim stirrups will fool a visual scale by at least ten pounds any day.

To continue the illusion of trimness, wear flowing fabrics that don't cling, and avoid very light, thin fabrics. Enjoy colors and prints, but shy away from the extremely large or shockingly loud patterns.

Properly fitted slacks, with a top tucked in and loosely bloused over can be more flattering than a large tunic, even if you have full hips. When selecting that top, remember medium size print patterns without much contrast in color make you appear smaller. If your bust is full, avoid bows, ruffles, pockets, and other designs that will draw unwanted attention and accent.

More than any other body type, the SOMETHING MORE woman needs to pay close attention to her accessories. Scarves, long strands of pearls, large earrings and pins—these are all designed just for YOU. Keep the size and scale of jewelry in balance with the silhouette of your outfit and body. Neck interest will draw the eyes to the face and away from the tummy and hips. Shoulder pads will add height and direct eyes upward. Bracelets, bangles, and rings attract eyes to the hands. Wear belts slung slightly lower, softly draped to one side, off-center.

Have fun with fashion! You DO have a choice to show off your own beauty and sense of self-confidence. Learn to translate your size into valuable self-worth with a positive attitude and a few wardrobe tips!

A LESSON FOR MID-LIFE

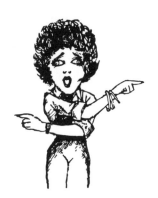

Wake up and smell the coffee, ladies! It's the real world out there, and NOBODY, not even Farrah Facett is perfect. She's growing older along with the rest of us, and from that ear-to-ear grin, she's sporting lately, she seems to be lovin' every minute of it. I know I am!

Approaching fifty (real soon now), I feel wonderful. Oh sure, I could lose ten pounds (Ok, Ok, so I could lose twenty pounds!). Definitely my hair would look more stylish without that little salt-and-pepper design, and of course, my eye shadow would be much smoother if there weren't those little creases across the lids. (Ever notice how it always seems to cake up right in that spot?)

Our culture creates the idea that beauty equates to love, that perfect image produces success, and the majority of us fall into the trap of believing everything depends on the approval of others. Our hopes, our dreams, and our expectations become geared to the way we THINK we must look.

Being thirty again is not on my list of top ten wishes. I'm proud and happy to be where I am. My children are almost raised (if they EVER completely are); I'm looking forward to grandchildren that I can spoil rotten (and then send home with their parents when the fun stops), and my house is paid for. I have no more PMS, and I finally qualified for a gold card before I'm eligible for membership in A.A.R.P. Life is grand!

At 175 pounds, I'm not obese—but I'm certainly not skinny. I occasionally think about dieting AGAIN, but I've finally convinced myself to accept ME for who I am. I spent almost twenty-five years of my life on a diet to maintain the slim chic image of a fashion maven. You name it; I tried it.

First it was easy losing five pounds whenever I wanted. Then it became ten, because with every loss, the weight would return two-fold. I found myself on a rotating diet plan trying every new gimmick or crazy scheme that was popular that week. I did Dexatrim, the wonder drug. This little colorful capsule could enable me to clean five houses, rake the yard, and paint somebody's barn—all before noon. On the white oblong pill Tenuate the feeling was less hectic but my heart beat fast, and I stayed awake for days on end.

At one of those diet places, I posed for their Before and After Plan; the problem was it wasn't long after before I was a larger version of BEFORE.

What am I forgetting? Oh yes, there was the place with the pre-packaged food. That I couldn't stomach; it tasted too much like plastic wrap it came stored in. (Frankly, the only thing that taste good out of a freezer is ice cream. Don't you agree?) I did spend six weeks once on Optifast Liquids. This hospital supervised health plan really worked. I lost 29 pounds in eight weeks, BUT I had no solid foods and the program cost about $425 per pound! Still I gained it all back plus, and they certainly didn't give me a refund for pounds added!

One of the best of the list is Weight Watchers. Although I have never been able to stick with the regimen, it does work and it is healthy. My only complaint is the weigh in sessions. I felt like a Catholic school girl at confession, falling on my knees and begging, "Forgive me, sisters, for I have sinned. His name is chocolate!"

Last but not least, I can't forget the revolving closet routine. I actually used to buy the same dresses in three sizes—a 8, a 10, and a 12. I thought if I always wore the same outfits, folks would say, "she hasn't gained weight; she's still wearing that same dress." Oh, what we won't do to fool our friends and feed our ego!

In the last few years, my life has taken on a whole new meaning as trivial things have been replaced with substance and importance. I no longer depend on looking in a mirror or zipping a perfect size 10 dress to make me happy. My joy comes from within, through the relationships I have with my family, my friends, and my God. I work hard to focus on the strengths of my life, not the weaknesses, concentrating on the good, not the bad.

Until I was forty. I really thought I HAD TO BE PERFECT! I guess I could try to blame that on my mother who worshipped and adored her only child and wanted her to grow up to be somebody, or I could say I needed to stay skinny because I owned a fashion boutique and customers expected the owner to have a modelish image or I could blame my husband who liked having a tall, slim younger (well, I am six years younger!) woman on his arm, or again I could go back and put the blame on society or magazine covers or movie stars or history or the Democrats (everyone blames them for something!), but it was ALL my fault. Unfortunately, it took a nervous breakdown, partially caused by the abuse of diet pills creating a chemical imbalance in my body to make me realize it was who I was, not how I looked that mattered.

Mother didn't care if I was a writer, a model, a homemaker, or waitress; she just loved me because I was her daughter. My customers weren't trying to look like me. Actually, shoppers are sometimes intimidated by sales clerks who are taller, thinner, or prettier than them. I certainly couldn't say I had an image to uphold for my store. People were there buying my service, my merchandise, my fashion knowledge, and convenient shopping—not my size 8 body.

And Larry... well,he probably would still like having a 120 lb. wife, but wouldn't every man? We have so many things to share, so many precious memories to build a life together on, that I couldn't ever imagine spending the rest of my life without him. Someday I can picture us sitting on the front porch in a swing recalling days long past. He'll turn to me and say, *"Remember the day Laura Lea went to kindergarten for the first time?"* (He won't say, *"and you looked fantastic in that red size 8 pantsuit."*) Then he might mention, *"What a great day it was when Billy graduated from college!"* (He won't say, *"and wow—that black and white fitted suit was great on you."*) Perhaps we'll shed a tear when he recalls, *"I'm so glad you were with me when we buried Meme."* (Not one mention of the size 9/10 navy blue Chanel suit!)

It took a painful mid-life lesson to make me realize the important little things in life. Of course, lipstick's nice, but a smile is much more important on your lips! Looking fabulous doesn't mean a thing if it's not accompanied by feeling fabulous! Life is meant to be enjoyed with and for the ones you love. Take time out to look in the mirror, check that smile, and you'll be perfect!!!

Sixty-Nine

HAIRDO HUES

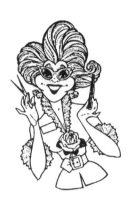

E ver wonder what your hair color has to say about your personality? A recent study by one of America's manufacturers of beauty products revealed some rather interesting, if not scientific data.

Let's start with brunettes. I'm one and have always liked my dark hair (even after the little wisps of white started creeping in.) The survey showed that brunettes were perceived as self-confident (that's me), sensual (that's me), sensitive (that's me), down-to-earth (that's me), and sultry (that's me!) Brunettes were more down-to-earth and less self-centered (77 and 47 percent, respectively) compared to blondes. They were more sultry (68 percent) and sensitive (79 percent) than redheads. (Wow, I like this survey, already!)

Results reflected that brunettes and redheads were considered more sympathetic by nature than blondes, and that redheads were definitely more aggressive and bolder than blondes and brunettes, put together!

There is a huge disagreement over who has more fun. Over 58 percent of all blondes swear they do, but so do brunettes and reds. On the self-confidence issue, 75 percent of brunettes said they see themselves in a positive light, while only 65 percent of blondes could say the same thing. Redheads soared ahead with 80 percent saying they were confident of their feelings of who and what they are as individuals.

Almost half (49 percent) of the blondes surveyed admit they consider themselves naive—and 50 percent of the other women agree. But only 25 percent of brunettes rated themselves naive, and redheads classified themselves as the savviest group with only 14 percent admitting feelings of naivete.

The color of woman's hair remains her most noticeable asset, affecting the way others perceive her, and the way she perceives herself. We tend to classify blondes as glamorous, redheads as temperamental, and brunettes as plain, but none of these theories apply. (In other words, forget the dumb blonde jokes. Odds are, she's not a true blonde anyway!)

For a few extra statistics on that special group of fair haired ladies, check out this profile from the survey:

❊ Percentage of women who have naturally blonde hair—16%

❊ Percentage who have brown or auburn hair—62%

❊ Percentage who have red hair—1%

The total number of gray hairs were not admitted to and were discreetly overlooked in this report, but the number of American women who color their hair is 35 million or 1/3 of the population! Of those the percentage who color blonde is 42%!

At what age do women start to color? For actual use of permanent dye, the average age is 36 years, but beginning with special effects and highlighting average is 27 years of age. It takes nine to twelve salon visits per year to keep up a double-process blonde color job for an average cost of $527 annually. The cost of maintaining blonde highlights for one year averages $750.

(Figures were not available on coloring hair brunette, red, or gray, but personally, I spend about $300 annually to keep the silver from shining through the dark brown!)

And so what difference does any of this make with the opposite sex?

Well, in the words of the ladies themselves:

✳ 91% of all blondes consider themselves popular with men.

✳ 74% of brunettes feel the same way.

✳ 64% of redheads felt they were popular.

Actually, despite what the surveys say (and remember, these were done by hair color companies), it's probably all in your head anyway—or on it!

CAN YOU BELIEVE WHAT YOU READ?

When I appeared in Little Rock, Arkansas, a reporter attended one of my fashion seminars and interviewed me for the Sunday edition of *The Arkansas Democrat* newspaper. A week or so later, one of my friends from that area called me almost in tears after seeing the headline which read: "She's not young; she's not pretty; she's not skinny..." I asked her to read on to the small print and she continued the article. Soon she admitted it was a great compliment. I was thrilled because the reporter described my life, my size, my looks, and how I managed to put it all together by creating a professional and personal image and lifestyle, despite those three strikes against me.

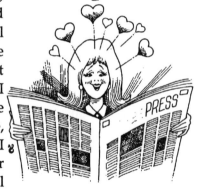

I am one of the lucky ones. Millions of American women view their physical being with disgust, and judge their entire social and professional success on how they look. Their physical and mental health is constantly threatened. Psychologists fight a seemingly unending battle against magazine covers and television images that daily try to convince us all that only the young, the tall, the thin can reach the heights of success, happiness, and true love.

A recent SELF magazine study revealed that 3/4 of the 9,000 women who responded to their survey said that their shape and weight were the most important factors in determining their feelings about their bodies. Twelve percent said they were extremely dissatisfied, sixteen percent were quite dissatisfied, twenty-five percent were just plain unhappy about the shape they were in. Each said this was in their thoughts constantly and had a disturbing effect on their daily life.

Tragically, it's getting to the point that American women are so obsessed over what's wrong with themselves—be it weight, shape, wrinkles, pimples, whatever—that they are failing to develop their potential as human beings. People with poor body image are so self critical, they usually fear rejection to such an extreme, they shy away from social situations, intimate relationships, and career opportunities. They throw health caution to the wind and take drastic measures to reshape their bodies and search for lost youth, no matter what the cost.

Blaming our age, our bodies, or even our circumstances for the failures and disappointments of life doesn't work. That's not what's wrong with life! Learn to accept yourself for who you are, physically and mentally. Develop a positive image of what you are and can become. (Notice, I did not mention DIET; life should not be lived without chocolate!)

Oh, back to the Arkansas story. The rest of that sentence in the fine print said, "She's not young; she's not pretty, she's not skinny.....she's just wonderful!" Even with three strikes against me, I hit a home run in that reporter's eyes. Show the world what really matters by being the best you can be with what God gave you!

WHAT'S IN A NAME?

A re you one of the almost 60 percent of the American population that is dissatisfied with your given name? Probably! I think every girl I ever met wished she were named something else—anything else, other than her own name. Perhaps this is a "southern thing," since female offspring below the Mason-Dixon line always are given double names, triple names, and worst of all—weird names, justified by the fact that these sacred names have been in the family for generations and must be passed down like heirlooms or fine china!

It has always been a bad habit that Southerners can't help but straddle their offspring with titles these children later try to forget, forge, or forsake. I think it affects women more than men, because young boys have a way of "losing" their formal names early in their childhood. William becomes Will or Billy; if he's William Robert, he's apt to quickly be tagged BILLY BOB. Richard is changed to Dick; Charles is Chuck. The male gender is so creative when it comes to nicknames; they answer to things like Bo, Tiger, Radar, Moose, and other strange animal titles. You need only look to today's headlines to see that in 1993 the leader of our country is not William Jefferson Clinton. To his family, he's Bubba; to his friends, he's Billy Jeff.

Unlike guys, girls are usually stuck with whatever name that's listed on their birth certificate. From the time I was old enough to understand words, I could never for the life of me, understand how my mother chose to label me: TOMMY JEAN FRANCES VAUGHAN. (Where was her mind on that fateful day in May 1945?) I used to pretend that the 23 letters were punishment for the 23 hours she spent in hard labor prior to bringing me into this world. Not so. Like all mothers, especially Southern ones, there was a meaning behind her madness.

She was one of seven children, and because my father was off fighting THE BIG ONE, WW II, she lived at home with her parents and siblings while awaiting my birth. There was only one other grandchild in the family then, so this pregnancy was regarded by all as something close to the second coming (or so the family story goes).

During the many hours proceeding my entry into this world, the rural hospital in McComb, Mississippi resembled a social gathering as my mother's relatives, friends, and their friends assembled to greet this long awaited new family member. The hours passed and the quiet watch turned into a party, an all night event with food, drink, and fun galore for all—my mother NOT included.

Leading the group were my Uncle Tommy (Thomas W. Beatty) who was my mother's older brother and closest friend, and my Aunt Sugar (Margarett Jean Beatty), her baby sister. They somehow became the lucky winners in the name lottery, and also doubled as my Godparents. Where the Frances came in is still a mystery, but it seems my grandmother thought it was a "pretty" name, and my grandmother ruled the roost. What she said was gospel, so it got thrown in at the last minute jut before the nurse completed the legal birth paperwork.

Remember Johnny Cash's song about "The Boy Named Sue?" You think HE had problems? Just try being the girl named Tommy. Everyone just assumes it's TOMMIE; they never ask; they just spell it that way—the feminine way. To get it corrected requires an explanation as to why I misspell my name. In person, this is an aggravation. In writing, it is a major undertaking! Computers, government agencies, even Ed McMahan is convinced I am Mr. Tommy Jean. Letters, messages, packages

Seventy-Six

come for the man of the house: Tommy! Telemarketers ask, "Is Mr. Tommy available, please?" I always answer, "He doesn't live here anymore." It's easier than explaining or listening to their sales pitch for life insurance or magazine subscriptions.

In 1963, I was drafted by Uncle Sam and received a very cordial letter saying my services were required for the Vietnam War. Can you imagine how much fun I had with that experience? Trying to convince the U.S. Government that I was really a girl was no easy task. I am sure to this day, there is someone in Washington who believes I was simply a draft dodger trying to avoid my manly duty.

(Think I could become President? Billy Jeff did!)

As a young teenager, I began to acquire nicknames, but none that really stuck, until that day my first employer said those magic letters, "T.J." It sounded so adult, so savvy, so hip in 1963 to be called T.J.

My mother immediately hated it. (I thought I might have to quit my part-time job.) My uncle didn't mind at all (he was a man—what did he care), but my Aunt Sugar... she was furious! (I never really understood why, since she didn't even use the name herself. Why should I have to carry it around for the both of us?) Our entire family knew her only as "Sugar," a name my grandfather gave her early in her childhood, and to strangers, she was just Margarett, no Jean added on. I was the one with the 23 letters, TOMMY JEAN FRANCES VAUGHAN!

By the time I opened my shop, the name change was easy. With the clothing store named T.J.'s... for Her, I soon became known to almost everyone (except my mother and my aunt), as T.J. My husband even took it one step further, affectionately shortening it to "Tee."

Even after all these years, I still have horror stories I can relate because of the Tommy name. I've been accused of trying to use my husband's credit card; I've been stopped from boarding a plane because they thought I was using someone else's ticket; and... oh, it just gets worse, I'd rather not go into the details.

The women's movement helped me tremendously as I was able to put a MS. in front of the Tommy and the T.J. I didn't, and don't consider it a slap in Larry's face or a denial of our marriage, because any time I use Mrs. Tommy, then I am considered to be Tommy's wife. (See you just can't win for losing in the name game!)

The one thing I vowed never to do was to burden a child of mine with a name he or she would not like. Growing up, I thought how silly it was that all girls from the South had to have double names, like all my cousins: Jocie Lea, Berta Jo, Barbara Sue, Ramona Ann, Elaine Kay, and even Vivian Jo Ann (another of those family triples!). Never ever, I swore, would I let this happen to a precious angel of mine. After all, I was a modern woman of the seventies; I had heard Helen Reddy roar!

Then in August of 1973 the big day came. Just like my mother some 28 years earlier, I spent over twenty hours in the hospital labor room before holding my beautiful, darling miracle of life in my arms. Suddenly, I wanted everyone around me to share in her love, and be a part of the celebration. A true good woman of the Confederacy, I returned to my roots, I followed my heritage and my heart and marked this child for life with a typical Dixie Double: the middle name of her grandmother, Mattie Lea, and the feminine version of her father's name, Lawrence. Combined with such thought and love, these two words spelled out LAURA LEA.

Thus another baby was brought into this world to grow up wondering how she would ever survive with such a name!

TRAVEL RIGHT TRAVEL LIGHT!

I am sure this title will bring a smile from anyone who has ever met me at the airport. On occasion, I have been known to get a little carried away when planning my travel wardrobe, but remember: Do as I say, not as I do! It is possible to survive three days with less than eight pair of shoes.

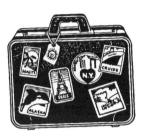

Seriously, I am getting better and am going to share some of my tips with those of you who may be spending time in the friendly skies. Don't expect my advice to resemble those *Traveler's Handbook* editions. I've read them all and disregarded almost everything they said. This should be fun, not a chore. Relax and enjoy the experience.

First, don't carry on baggage; I check my luggage. Maybe it's a feminine thing or part of that Southern Belle complex, but I don't like dragging heavy garment bags and suitcases through airports. Have you ever been fortunate enough to find a flight that goes anywhere without changing planes in Atlanta, Dallas, or Chicago? (I am sure on the way to heaven, there's a stopover AND a vehicle change at O'Hare!) If you have to walk the terminals, do it without the extra forty pounds. I like to arrive rested and ready to enjoy my new surroundings.

With the recent down-sizing of airplanes, it is next to impossible to find empty overhead storage areas for carry-ons, so I end up as the person who has to straddle two bags and a briefcase while my chin rests on my knee caps. This makes for a real pretty sight when lunch is delivered.

Seventy-Nine

My bottom line suggestion: Check 'em! According to my Delta frequent flier records, I have flown 532,653 air miles in the last three years (just on their planes), give or take a mile or two. I'm not about to figure out how many trips or segments that is, but I can honestly say, I HAVE NEVER LOST A PIECE OF LUGGAGE! (I promise; I swear: I knock on wood!) I have had three or four bags delayed, no more than three hours, perhaps twice, but that's it, so how can it make sense to risk life and limb performing manual labor through airports. That's what skycaps are for. Be sure to tip a minimum of $1.00 total, or fifty cents per bag, and these professionals will make sure your luggage is directed to the right location. (It doesn't hurt to double check the destination tags AND to over tip a little bit. Remember my track record? It works, I'm living proof!)

Even if you aren't having to carry that bag yourself, there is no reason to take along the whole house for a simple three day getaway. This is not one of those times when more is less, but when smaller is best. I have all my cosmetics in the sample sizes for travel. No one needs a six month supply of cleansing cream or a 14 oz. hairspray. By purchasing everything in trial size containers and refilling them when empty, I am actually able to carry all these items in my handbag. (This is especially wonderful for flight delays or for a quick fix-up just prior to landing!)

Most of my garments are rolled for packing. I have found it is much easier to lay several items on top of each other across the bed, then fold sleeves and pant legs across and loosely roll up. The real professional packers recommend placing tissue paper or plastic cleaner bags between these folds, but I seldom take the time. I've found the wrinkles quickly fall out as soon as items are hung (if you unpack upon arrival!). I carry a small can of WRINKLE FREE spray for touchups, but hanging garments on the shower rod and allowing the hot water to steam will usually solve any problems.

Eighty

If necessary, even the most economical hotels have complimentary irons that can be sent up from housekeeping. Leave those bulky household items at home, and pack that great pair of yellow pumps instead! (Housekeeping can't furnish those!)

In the FASHION section I discuss travel packing for accessories. This is a must for me, as my definition of changing outfits is sometimes just switching earrings and shoes. Those handy little divided pouches and roll-ups will keep everything neat and untangled. On occasion, when I plan my entire trip's daily ensembles, I will package the co-ordinating accessories in individual ziplock bags. It makes them easy to find without worrying what goes with what today. (I am told Hillary Clinton has a wardrobe consultant who does this for each of her outfits. The accessories are packaged and attached to the hanger of the appropriate costume.) Pantyhose are also best stored in individual baggies or a zippered lingerie case with clear pockets. Shoe bags will protect your footwear from scuffing against each other and from staining your clothing.

I suggest you pack an ample supply of empty plastic bags for dividing soiled and clean clothes for the return trip, as well as for damp swimwear. I carry an extra little fold-up tote bag inside my luggage, because I never fail to come home with more goodies than I started with. Allow space for those souvenirs or that fabulous bulky sweater you found that couldn't be left in Cleveland!

One of the best lessons I've learned from carrying my own bags is to divide and conquer! Two medium bags are much much easier to handle than one large. Soft side luggage is lighter and seems to withstand the rough treatment of baggage claim better than the more structured hard pieces. Label each piece with your name and home address, and the place you will be staying in your designated city. For extra precaution, include just

Eighty-One

inside the top of your suitcase a copy of your personal information as well as a travel itinerary. Should your luggage accidently be picked up by someone else by mistake, it can easily be returned to you on your trip without any delay. If your luggage is just the ordinary basic issue (and it should be—don't waste your money trying to impress fellow travelers or hotel bellmen), I suggest you identify it with a stripe or ribbon or something special. All suitcases look alike when that thing starts going round. It's easy for me to take a seat and tell the skycap, "The ones with the black and white polka dot ribbons!" (Now don't you use that, we'll get our bags mixed up!)

Notice I said, "Sit down and wait for the bags." You'll find after awhile that travel has to be relaxing and fun, or it'll kill ya! I try to treat each trip as a new adventure to be experienced to the fullest. Again, I disregard most of the travel advice that I read in magazines. I absolutely hate it when someone recommends "Dress comfortably; wear a warmup and tennis shoes."

A DC-9 is not a gym or a health club! Would you go to the office in a tank top and shorts? Are you planning on a heavy workout involving exercise and perspiration? Then leave those things at home.

A professional should look the role, whether in a boardroom or a boarding room. A comfortable pants suit or soft skirt and blouse will look nice and no one will mistake you for Richard Simmons. (I once flew in the seat across from him on a flight from New Orleans to Los Angeles. He's a delightful man, and he actually had on that little blue nylon tank and those short silky stripe shorts. I expected him to break into "Sweatin' with the Oldies" at any time, but let's not forget: This is his professional wardrobe, so he was dressed correctly... I guess.)

Eighty-Two

The old saying, "You never have a second chance to make a first impression," applies to travel as well as every other situation in life. On many occasions I have noticed passengers being treated in direct relation to the way they are dressed. You'll get better service, bigger smiles, and more peanuts in a business suit than in denim cutoffs and a crop top. I dress prepared for an overbooked economy section, hoping for an upgrade. I learned a long time ago when the best seats get changed around, they are given to the best dressed! It's worth wearing a blazer to end up sipping Diet Coke out of a real crystal glass in First Class.

Whether you travel once a week or once a year, there's no reason to do it yourself. Travel agents are at your disposal, free of charge. Their commissions are paid by the airlines, hotels, and rental car companies, so why should you bother calling around to find the best rates and flight schedules. Contact your local friendly agent and hand the duties over to them. In almost all cases, you'll find these people are looking out for your best interests, and will locate you the best prices available. They want your business. Compare and shop around; ask your friends. This is one less hassle for you, leaving more time for the important things in life, like bubble baths, chocolate candy, or just taking a deep breath!

For those of you who can't believe a "Travel" article would be in the FUN section, I have to admit, when I am off the road and not working, one of my main pleasures in life is travel. My bags are always ready! Where ya want to go?

Eighty-Three

EVERYBODY
LOVES A SALE!

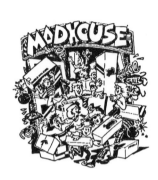

After reviewing the subjects I had included in the FUN section, I soon noticed it was almost all FASHION. AT first, I panicked and returned to the typewriter to do a re-write; then I realized this is FUN to me, and most of the women I know. "Shop til ya drop" may be an adage left over from the 1980's, but "Buy what ya can" is still one of the great pleasures of a lady's life.

A shopping trip can be a chore or a fun expedition, depending on how you view your life, your body, and the current amount of your Visa balance. Personally, I LOVE a sale! Just seeing those three little words, "Reduced for Clearance" will make my heart beat faster. If you are also one of those folks whose blood pressure rises at the sight of yellow tags with slash marks and numbers that end in $.99, read on for your own safety sake.

The wise consumer is one who plans ahead, sets goals, defines a wardrobe, and is not swayed by the yellow polka dot to-die-for blouse that will match absolutely nothing in her closet. You can be one of these savvy shoppers by learning how to recognize when a sale is really a sale, and when a bargain is actually a good buy. (There is a definition I once read, "A bargain is anything that doesn't fit!")

The best times to get true values on clothing are January and July. This is, of course, when store owners are having to clear out merchandise to make room for the next season's goodies. Actually, this has no relationship to reality, because just as it gets cold enough to wear a sweater, the local department store is selling out of them. The day before your summer vacation, every swimsuit in the place is on the discount table. (All the tops are sized large and the bikini bottoms are marked extra-small!) This is not real life; it's the fashion world—and you can be the beneficiary of the local shop owner's misfortune if you play your cards right!

Stick with shops and department stores that you are familiar with. If you are a regular customer (or at least visitor), you can compare merchandise and prices; you can keep your eye out for that special group of sweaters or that special dress that should go on the markdown rack soon. Drop by frequently to check out new arrivals, and note the selling progress on the items you're hoping will go down in price before your resistance wears down.

By trying on garments earlier in the season, it is possible to determine if something is oversized or cut smaller. (This is often the reason for many markdown items. They simply were never tried on in the correct size.) Another reason for these advance try-on sessions is to avoid the dressing room rush on the actual first sale day. If you know what you're after in the correct size and section, even an overflow crowd of crazed sale shoppers won't put a dent in your style! (Remember those cartoons of women ripping slacks in half because there was only *one* size 14 in blue. In my store, these scenes actually happened. Try to get in and out and without any bruises or serious injuries!)

There are many trendy items that can not be considered a deal even at 75% off. (Forget the glitzey jewel sweater or the gold trim ankle pants with the fringe on the hip pockets!) Avoid purchasing garments that are this year's fad and next year's folly. Swimsuits, classic apparel, basic blouses, cardigans, turtlenecks, and outerwear seldom change drastically from one season to the next.

Eighty-Five

Concentrate on spending the bulk of your sale allowance in these areas. Steer clear of anything that requires alterations or weight loss. (This will be one of those things you'll put in the rummage sale three years from now, with the tags still in tact.)

As a former specialty shop owner, I know who got the best buys in my store: the regular customers! Form a relationship with a sales assistant in your favorite boutique. She'll be delighted to complete a reference card listing your favorite brands, colors, and sizes. When you make a major purchase, she'll record it and note that you need additional pieces to round out your wardrobe. Having someone who cares about you is the best way to be assured of first choice on the reduced merchandise. (She'll probably put it in the back before it ever hits the sale rack.) Tell her when you particularly like an item but are unable to pay the regular price. Mention you'd like to have these slacks *"if they are ever reduced."* Even when sales people are not working on commission, they still want happy satisfied customers. Their success comes from moving merchandise; I promise they'll get in touch. Put your name on their mailing list. Better yet, give 'em your number! (Don't wait on the U.S. mail.)

If all this sounds too calculated and planned, then you are truly one of those women who gets her kicks from S-A-L-E! If you can afford it, I say "Go for it!" If not, leave the Visa card and checkbook at home. Allot yourself a limited amount of spendable cash, and head to the mall for a great time!

P.S. Don't overlook the fact that most final clearance items come with a tag that reads: ALL SALES FINAL—NO RETURNS.

SECTION III

FEELINGS

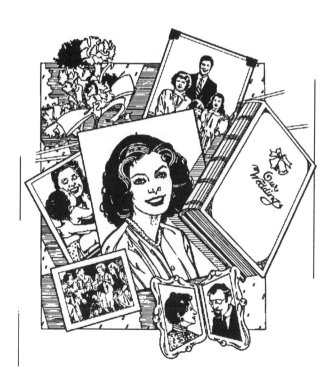

FEELINGS....

*"*Feelings, nothing more than feelings..." Did you know that's one of the top three songs requested each and every night in piano bars across the country? There's always someone out there trying to remember or forget or just make sense of it all.

For most of my adult life, I've either written down my thoughts on yellow note pads, typed them out, or just recently began putting them into computer. It isn't exactly a journal or diary—it's just how I feel about TODAY. Doogie Howser, M.D. has nothing on me; I was just a little before my time. Too bad, it could've made a great television series, T. J. Reid—Woman.

The first years I can't seem to locate. I guess most of them have been lost, thrown out, or hidden away. When the children were young, I wrote them very personal letters on the pages of their baby books, and I have these carefully stowed away for them to have after I'm gone. (As when I die,—not when I go to Seattle!)

Of the thoughts I could find, I put together about thirty days that were special to me, days when either life, government, fashion, home, children, friends, media, or God gave me reason to ponder the future of womankind. Some are happy days remembering my children and their accomplishments; some are mad days when I wanted to beat up on somebody; many are sad days when I just wanted to sit down and cry. For some reason, tears never came without putting the thoughts on paper; tempers weren't calmed unless I dealt with it in print, and joys seemed so much more pleasurable when I remembered them in words.

This is what I share with you. The fashion you've seen; the fun you've read; here are the feelings.

Eighty-Eight

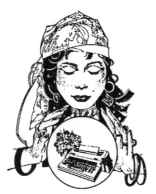

WHEN I GROW UP TO BE A WRITER

Even though I dearly love my store and being a "fashion maven," sometimes late at night when I come down here to this typewriter, I wonder what if... what if I had become a writer instead of opening the store. What if I had published that great American novel, written that prize-winning poem, been the toast of Broadway with that dramatic play? I guess at 35, I'm a little old to be doing what ifs, but still... maybe someday.

I can't ever remember a time when I didn't want to be a writer, or a fashion designer, or an artist. My grandmother, JoJo, used to go to work from 4 A.M. til 2 p.m., so in the mid-afternoon she usually tried to lie down and rest for a couple of hours before fixing supper. Unfortunately, she seldom ever got that rest. All my early years, beginning as soon as I could walk and talk, were spent with pen and paper, flopping all over her featherbed, saying, "Look here, Jojo."

By the time I reached first grade, I could not only write my ABC's; I could spell, rhyme, sketch, and quote the

Bible. Thanks to this precious lady and her afternoon naps, in 1951 I was just about ready to be published! But it took nine years to happen.

She was the happiest person in the whole wide world that day in 1960 when my first acceptance letter arrived. Yes, ME—little old me, a fifteen year old kid with a typewriter in Kentwood, Louisiana was having a short story published in a national magazine in New York. She carried that HEP CAT teen magazine around for years, forcing friends and strangers to read the talents of her grandchild. She'd tell them all about the $50 check, and how it was just the beginning of a career that would surpass John Steinbeck and Tennessee Williams, for sure. She wasn't proud or anything; she was just a grandmother.

When I opened my dress shop, she was equally proud; maybe I'd be a designer and those sewing lessons she gave me would finally pay off. At least I wasn't gonna have to cook and clean; that was her main concern. I wasn't raised to do that, she'd say, "You're too smart not to make something of yourself." Little did she realize the importance of her life's vocation. Long after her death, folks for miles around still bragged about Mrs. Beatty's cakes and her chicken pie. Nothing tasted better than her hot rolls on a cold winter's day, and no one would ever consider getting married without one of Mrs. Beatty's three-tier wedding bakery delights. The Kentwood football team for decades, never took the field without first chowing down on one of her special pre-game roast beef and potato meals. It was the food that inspired champions, and made a community, and its residents, love her.

Cooking, clothing, writing, I guess they all can make a difference. It just depends on who's doing what and whether they enjoy doing it. JoJo L-O-V-E-D to cook; that made her happy. Maybe one day, I'll write a book just for her. That'd make me happy!

Ninety

PREPPIE COWGIRLS

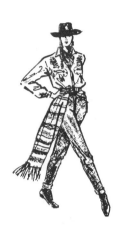

As the fashion guru of the community, I always try my best to keep everyone up on the latest in the fashion world, but this season it's no easy feat determining the fine line between fashion and fad. It's gonna be up to each individual's own taste and budget to decide what best fits their 1981 lifestyle.

For example, there are two very different and distinct extremes happening in apparel this season. It's the year of the preppies (a return to the classics of the 1955-65 era), and the time of the urban cowgirl (God bless John Travolta and that bucking bull at Gilley's). To be on the safe side, one can cover both of these trends by adding just a few simple extra items to their wardrobe:

(1) A Button-down oxford shirt with a monogram (preferably your own initials)

(2) A suede vest (with or without fringe)

(3) A pullover knit shirt (alligator required!)

(4) A wide leather belt with a name embossed on the back (again, it's best if it's YOUR name.)

(5) A pair of jeans with a name on the back pocket (In this instance, it should NEVER be your name!)

(6) A pair of walk shorts (No name required anywhere)

To top off this country/classic look you'll need two types of footwear: a pair of top-siders and cowboy boots. Then the real test of your fashion know-how is understanding which of these pieces to wear with which! Good luck!

Ninety-One

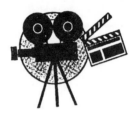

What Makes a Movie Critic?

Did you ever notice if a movie wins an Academy Award, you probably didn't like it? I sometimes wonder where they get their voters, and who in the world thinks these disasters are worth applauding.

I did enjoy seeing "On Golden Pond"; it was a truly beautiful and touching motion picture, but Fonda and Hepburn certainly didn't deserve Academy Awards for their performances. How hard could it have been for them to play themselves—just two old people? There were so many other actors much more deserving.

If you're planning on rushing out to see "Chariots of Fire," let me save you some money up front. Pay attention, I'm trying to be a true friend. This was the slowest, most boring, badly acted, and poorest photographed movie I have ever sat through in my life. The popcorn was even stale! Go out and buy the album; the only thing that's any good is the sound track, and music, a movie does not make.

If I leave a theater with tears streaming down my cheeks, I always feel a deep satisfaction that I've gotten my money's worth. If (as Larry swears) I judge a movie by the amount of Kleenex I need for the ending, then "Officer and A Gentlemen" is certainly a four tissue event.

Rough language and sizzling sex qualify this film for a heavy R rating, but the boot camp talk is realistic, and I expect Richard Gere to rate an R, even when he's fully dressed. (He's always been a favorite of mine, but he's about to lose his place to that new kid, Tom Cruise!)

The love story ending of "Officer" sends you home with a warm happy feeling that any romantic fool will adore. Don't be embarrassed to applaud the ending; I did! (Larry was!)

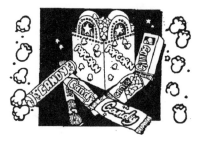

The Windsong Man

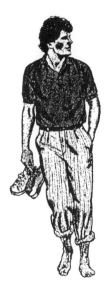

Today is August 13, 1981; it's simply just Thursday to most people in the world, but to Laura Lea, it is "only five more days til her birthday." We began this daily countdown about three weeks ago, and have faithfully been informed every time the number changes. Gosh, it's hard to believe she'll be eight years old... and Billy is seventeen, a senior in high school this year. When did I get so old?

Last week I was forced to realize my age when I decided I needed to read *Seventeen*, young America's favorite magazine, or so they advertise themselves. I figured I should keep up with the latest news on teens if I wanted to cultivate this junior customer in my store. Anyway, no explanation needed; I just wanted to read *Seventeen*.

I was delightfully surprised by the excellent choice of articles, poetry, and features. Even the ads seemed more interesting and alive than in the more mature adult things I read like *Cosmo* or *Redbook*. One thing for certain, these publishers know who spends the money in America. Of the 362 pages in *Seventeen*, over 200 of them were full page advertisements disguised as fun reading, while the other 162 pages contained at least several subtle mentions of some product or another. This consumer syndrome thing starts early in life, doesn't it? From the cradle to the grave, you better believe there's always gonna be somebody out there trying to sell you something. (If Laura Lea only knew how great it was to be seven years, eleven months, and twenty-five days old!)

The one thing I couldn't turn away from in *Seventeen* was the Windsong ad. I stopped to drool, as always. It brought back memories of many years ago when as a teenager myself, I would faithfully clip out his picture every month and pin it to the wall by my bed. (The Windsong guy was always a HUNK, even back then.} Each and every morning, I awoke face-to-face with this handsome man whispering softly, "Can't seem to forget you. Your Windsong stays on my mind."

Some things never change, whether it's 1961 or 1981. The fashions on the pages are still classic; the shirts are again buttoned-down, the skirts are getting shorter, and the Windsong man is still gorgeous! (Maybe even cuter than Tom Cruise...No, I don't think so!)

WHO'S MINDING THE STORE?

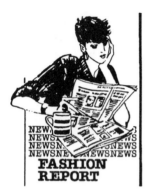

FASHION REPORT

"Be Dazzled in Dallas" was what all the market brochures promised. So I'm off on my annual holiday buying trip for the shop. Seems sort of stupid buying Christmas clothes in August, but that's the way it works in the fashion biz. For this Christmas, I'm already seeing samples of lurex sweaters, rhinestone trimmed hosiery, shiny things to light up your life. We may even need sunglasses for some of this stuff!

My mother worries each and every time I fly, but not me; I love it. Still, I must admit I did have second thoughts this time because of the air controller's strike. (I wish Ronald Reagan had just stayed a movie actor! What a mess he seems to be making of things.)

Anyway, I boarded the plane off to Big D, and all was going just fine. After my complimentary orange juice and blueberry muffin, I decided to leisurely flip through the airline magazine to finish off the last fifteen minutes of the trip prior to landing. The first article I turned to announced, "Dallas-Fort Worth Airport is the third busiest in the U.S. Twelve major airlines provide more than 1,000 daily arrivals and departures from this busy field."

Who thought this was news I wanted to read TODAY? My mind did some very quick calculating, and I immediately began to wonder who is minding the store down there in the control room, while the real pros are out on the picket line? What were the odds of us making it down alive if 40,333 planes were landing and taking off in a one hour period? I prayed someone down there had binoculars, and someone up high was watching over us.

Make a note in memo book: Never read freebie magazines on airplanes!

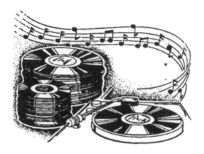

One is Not A Lonely Number

G rowing up as an only child, I was alone a lot of the time, but not lonely—just alone. There is a big difference, and I enjoyed it thoroughly. Those were the times I spent learning to read, write, and draw. The hustle and bustle of my household today is sometimes just too much for me, so I relish the wee hours of the morning when I can slip down the stairs to my private hideaway office with this keyboard as my only company. (Does that sound strange to you?) It probably does to most normal people, but I crave that peace and quiet sometimes.

Last week on the way to the airport I again realized how much I enjoy my own company. I spent that entire uninterrupted hour just riding along listening to WYNK and traveling in my own private world. I caught myself laughing out loud at some of the stupid song lyrics, and turned quickly to make sure no one in the passing cars had been watching me.

Country music songs are really getting to the point of ridiculous now days. Did you ever actually listen to the words and the stories they tell? Country queen Tammy

Wynette wasn't content with giving us "D-I-V-O-R-C-E" and "Stand By Your Man." Her latest tear jerker is " Cowboys Don't Shoot Straight Like They Used To," with the flip side, "He's Rolling Over in Someone Else's Clover." I swear to God, that's the real title!

Glen Campbell, my one-time favorite, had two of his old songs played in the last hour. Larry and I went to his concert on our first date, but he's changed now. GLEN—not Larry! I think I liked him better before he stole sweet Sara from Mac Davis, became a rhinestone cowboy, and then dumped her for femme fatale, Tanya Tucker. *PEOPLE* magazine recently described Tanya's new wardrobe as "Fredericks of Nashville." To me, it looks like she's just showing up in her underwear.

KIDS CLOTHES VS. SCHOOL BOARD

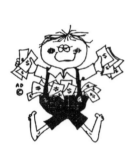

I know I am an info-maniac. I read five newspapers every day, watch the six o'clock and ten o'clock news faithfully, read about forty magazines a month, and several books. I just can't seem to fill my head with enough useless trivia, I guess. Still I do find out some interesting and amazing things. All this reading and working keeps me away from the typewriter lately, but today I read something I couldn't let go unmentioned.

I can not believe with all the hunger, child abuse, rape, and murder going on in this world, that the latest national news is about the bickering between some teacher and parent group over the effect of designer label clothing on a child's mental well being. It seems there is a "We're Special, Too" group formed to help ban designer garments from our children's wardrobes, thus removing any social or status symbol barriers which may or may not be warping youngsters' mental attitudes.

Can you believe this? Will it soon apply to adults, too? Are we going to have national uniforms to wear each day? Kids are being beaten up, murdered, and God knows what else; twenty-five percent of all eighth graders can't read, and these people who claim to be highly educated mentors have nothing better to do than go out on the playground to count Calvins and Izods.

One Hundred

Don't they realize these are the same kids who'll grow up and be comparing cars and boats and stereo systems with their neighbors in the subdivisions? What'll we do then, ban Cadillacs and put everyone in a Ford Escort?

The old adage will always be true, *"The only difference in men and boys is in the price of their toys."* Don't be messing with my kid's toys or his pants!

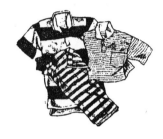

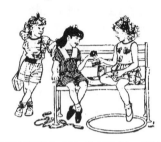

THE PAIN OF
PARENTHOOD

I t's been quite a while since I've been down here writing, but it's been a busy time at the store; my life feels like it's in overdrive half the time. I'm just too exhausted at night. My writing urges come in spurts, governed mostly by my mood swings. (Wonder if F. Scott Fitzgerald ever suffered from P.M.S.? I know Lewis Grizzard does!)

I've been under a great deal of pressure since Christmas. If you're a parent, you'll understand my pain when I confess that we did not have an ATARI. (There, I've finally said it aloud to the world.) I must admit, it was rough going for a few months. Laura Lea lamented daily as to her shameful state, reminding us almost hourly that WE were (without any doubt) the ONLY family in the entire city of Amite without electric pac-men running through the six o'clock news. How embarrassing it was for her!

Since her birthday last week and her ATARI "surprise" gift (she only asked for it three hundred and ten times!), I can again walk down the street with my head held high, secure in the knowledge that we have been able to keep up with the Joneses, ...or at least with Angie, Paula, and Cindy of the fourth grade.

One Hundred Two

A WOMAN VICE-PRESIDENT????

W hat's the old expression, "If the shoe fits, wear it?" Well, that's certainly appropriate for this week's news, but I'm not really sure how I feel about this.

I'm not as liberal as I sometimes appear, and I'm also not convinced Geraldine is who I want as the next vice-president. It'll do wonders for the Mondale election ticket, because I don't know anyone, who knows anyone, that likes Mondale. Do you? Still, to vote for her just because she's a woman is not a legitimate reason either. On the other hand, she is prettier than George Bush, and since the V.P. serves no real purpose in government anyway, why not let her go for it. It's a giant step for womanhood, or should I say personhood? I never know what's proper these days since we're all so genderless.

If it's all the same with the women-libbers, I'm gonna continue to ride the fence on some of these issues. Personally, I like being a woman—not a person. I enjoy doors being opened, hands being held, and most important of all: Gas tanks being filled! As the title of that great American classic reads, "Real Women Don't Pump Gas," and I don't. Sometimes I'll run the car until it's almost on empty or get on and off the interstate ramp in three different towns, but I'm gonna find me a place that is full-service. I just can't bring myself to do it. It's a Southern Belle thing.

There are a lot of things I can accomplish, and I'm extremely proud of them, but Larry knows I don't open jars, pop pop-tops, light the furnace, program the VCR, or carry out the garbage. I hope Geraldine and her feminist

One Hundred Three

buddies don't mess up any of the good things I have going in my life!

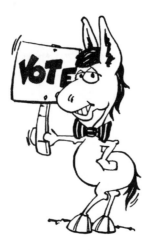

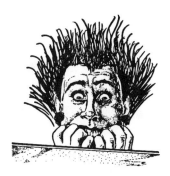

What A Mess I'm In

I just picked up a copy of *New Woman* magazine, and although I don't always agree with their editorial policy, all in all it's a pretty good read. The April issue is excellent with several articles on stress, one "Slowing Down in the Fast Lane," and another "Stress for Success." They seem to be condoning two entirely different theories, but both were interesting and gave me something to read while trying to eliminate stress in my life. There were tests to determine your stress level and individual problem areas, so I decided to take the sample quiz. I found out, unfortunately, I died two years ago!

I know I need to lose weight and shape up, but even though the body is willing, the mouth is still open. I can't seem to get started on any kind of diet plan. Actually, I've had enough of those to last a lifetime. Maybe I'll just try prayer. There's a new Weight Watcher's version that recently came out. It goes:

"Dear Lord, If I can't be thin, please make all my friends be fat!"
That pretty much sums up how I feel about the situation.

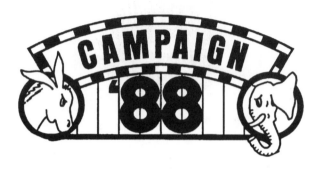

Am I Really A Democrat?

Never discuss sex, religion, or politics with friends. I've heard that all my life, but I'm still too stupid to listen. I need to talk to someone soon before this Presidential election date. I'm feeling a little unsure of myself, my beliefs, my party—everything.

Yet, I remember I once read: "If one is not a liberal at 20, he has no heart. If one is not a conservative at 40, he has no head." I don't recall, but I bet some politician made that statement, and it only makes me feel more confused. I am forty; that just might justify why as a life-long Democrat, my greatest fear at this moment is Michael Dukakis as President.

Christmas '88

W hat a fabulous holiday we had this year! Our house stayed full of rotating guests, and we seem to run an airport shuttle every day or so as folks were flying in and out so fast I could barely keep the linens changed.

Since Billy couldn't come home until the 23rd, we decided to wait and put up our tree then. It really seemed strange not having a dead tree on the 27th of December. We are so accustomed to putting it up so early, they're usually straw by Christmas Eve. This one could've lasted well into February if I had left it up.

It was a different kind of holiday season for us. The children kept busy with their friends, all heading in different directions to their own parties and events. Billy and his old high school buddy, Scott, played a few rounds of golf this week, and even that seemed odd to me. I kept remembering them with their tennis rackets and those daily practices all through the years. Has it really been ten years since we sat and watched them in the state playoffs?

What a depressing thought! Yes, this is a Christmas when age is creeping up on me. I felt so much older as I hung those stockings. Of course, as Santa, I was still there to fill them, but now it's with make up, cassette tapes, golf balls, and of course, dollar bills. Their idea of a wonderful Christmas Eve was riding around town in the Mustang with the top down, while they were freezing under blankets. No more dolls or toy trucks under the tree.

It's sort of sad to realize they're all grown up; sad, but wonderful, too. I've seen them spread their wings and grow from that tiny 20-inch baby boy to that handsome 6'1" young man already on his way up the corporate ladder, and from that chubby bouncing tot to that thin, sophisticated teenage miss with such high hopes and dreams sparkling in her bright eyes.

Enough of this... Soon I'll be singing, "Sunrise, sunset." Hand me the Kleenex, please.

What did I get for Christmas this year? My gift to me was a subscription to *"How to be Fabulous at 40!"* How could I resist buying it? Ed McMahon said I'd win ten million dollars just for sending in the card. (By the way, when he calls, I'll give you the subscription, I'll take the cash. With that kind of money, who needs fabulous and who cares about 40?) .

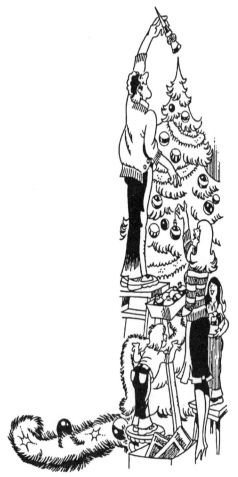

One Hundred Eight

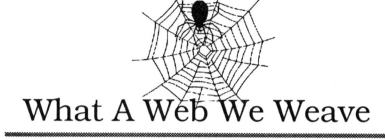

What A Web We Weave

L arry has been so wonderful about all the traveling I am having to do as I build this new and different career. Most husbands would never stay home alone for days on end, cook their own meals, and put up with a mad woman who locks herself up in a room late at night and types away on the typewriter til morning light. He is a dream, and he's supporting me as I try to get on paper, *WHAT MOTHER NEVER TOLD YA BOUT RETAIL...* the small store survival guide. It's shaping up, at last.

The gift that Larry gave me last week brought tears to my eyes and joy to my heart. (No matter how mad he makes me, he has a way of turning on the charm!) I was working late as always preparing to take yet another plane to another far away location. He leaned over as I sat in the middle of the bedroom floor sorting clothes for the trip, and he handed me a box from the jewelry store. I immediately thought, "Diamonds, silver—he knows winters don't wear gold!" But, alas it was gold, the ugliest gold pin I believe I've ever seen, until I realized IT was a spider! (That's Larry's nickname!)

He sweetly kissed me and said, "Now wear this everywhere you go, and I'll always be looking over your shoulder." Is that SPECIAL or what? How can I help but love this man?

To answer your curiosity: When Larry was eighteen or so, he and another guy went to try to join the Army. At the headquarters they were told to strip for their physicals and wait in a room for the medics. Larry was, at the time, about 5'8' and weighed maybe 120 pounds (if he had just finished off a full glass of water). The other boy was a towering fellow hitting the scales at close to 300 pounds.

When the doctor walked in, he looked up in shock, and said, "My God, they're sending me spiders and elephants now!"

I don't really know whatever happened to the other guy, but Larry has been called SPIDER ever since!

If you see me around, look for the spider. I now have at least twenty of them. (People send them to me in the mail all the time.) You can just about bet that I'll have one sitting atop my shoulder standing guard for the day!

One Hundred Ten

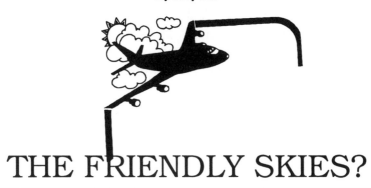

THE FRIENDLY SKIES?

I always fly Delta, BUT... on 2/15/89 I was forced to spend a day on Northwest Airlines. You know the commercial? It has the pleasant voice that says, "Northwest, look to us," and the happy fliers are going off into the sunset. Don't believe a word; it ain't necessarily so!

This particular week I was forced to change a reservation to Arkansas because the entire state was one big sheet of ice. They aren't accustomed to 8 degree temperatures. The day I finally got to travel turned out to be Ash Wednesday... Yes, like a fool I was in the New Orleans Airport the day AFTER Mardi Gras, the single largest holiday of the year for this party town. That alone qualifies me for admission to an insane asylum, but let me go on; it gets much worse.

The ticket agent was amazed that some idiot in their computer system had allowed me to change my non-refundable, non-changeable ticket just because of a little bad weather, and he proceeded to give me a lecture about it. Little did he realize, he had picked the wrong person on the wrong day in the wrong place, and I let him have a piece of my mind. Hopefully one I won't miss! After our little discussion, he handed me my tickets and I stomped off!

One Hundred Eleven

On the first leg of my trip, I was in a center seat between two robust men, just over the wing section. Even though the engine noise was extremely loud, one of the men wanted to tell me his life story (and from what I could barely hear, he hadn't had a fun time). I finally got him to stop when I offered him a part of my USA TODAY. It took him longer to get through one page than it took me to read an entire section. Not that I'm calling him slow or anything, but we should all be afraid. This man sells medical equipment for life saving situations in trauma units!

Delta has me spoiled with their cute, perky, friendly flight attendants, so the girls at Northwest came as quite a surprise. Those poor darlings must have a very different job application to complete. They resembled the before of makeover advertisements and were dressed in wine uniforms with gold braid and buttons. I feel sure they were bought at an excellent price because it's the same outfit that all bellmen at the Marriott wear, and waiters at the Sheraton.

When asked what beverage I preferred, I automatically said, "diet Coke," to which she replied, "No mam, we got Pepsi." I said, "OK, How about 7-Up?" She said, "No mam, we got Sprite." I said, "Then I'll take Dr. Pepper." She said, "No mam, we got ginger ale." By then the rest of the passengers were getting restless and thirsty, so I said, "Well, then I'll just have grapefruit juice." She answered, "No mam, we got orange." "OK,OK,OK, I'll take it!" At this moment I began to have some serious doubts about my chances of arriving in Memphis, much less further on to Little Rock. I could just imagine her on the microphone saying. "No mam, this is Omaha."

Changing planes in Memphis turned out to be a foot race. I had to walk from the end of terminal C to the end of terminal A while dragging two bags of accessory samples, my handbag, and my heavy winter coat. (Remember this

One Hundred Twelve

is February.) It was somewhere near Gate B-22 that I realized this Arkansas client wasn't paying me nearly enough for this job. I made a mental note to raise the fee on arrival.

The group waiting to go on to Little Rock looked much better than the left-over Mardi Gras crew in New Orleans. Everyone was wide awake and not one single person had on a stupid hat, was holding a Pat O'Brien's glass, or throwing up in the corner of the concourse. What a relief!

The DC 9 plane from Memphis to Little Rock had 22 rows of seats in economy class with a total seating for about a hundred passengers. We were a small group boarding, but guess where my seat was? You got it.... 22C! That little guy at the counter in New Orleans had won again. He might've given me a ticket, but he made darn sure I regretted every mile of it.

Sitting in the rear of an airplane means two things: You're the last one to get served, and you have a perfect view of everyone who has to use the restroom. I fooled them on the serving part, because I bought my own Diet Coke during my hike from Terminal C to Terminal A. My main problem for the moment was luggage. I suddenly realized: If he had made my life this miserable in the air, where had he sent my suitcases?

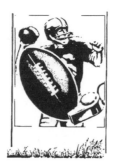

Farewell, Tom Landry,
My Old Friend

The guy on the TV just said, "Wake up, it's March 4th and 5:30 A.M., Good Morning Houston!" What a wonderful time to be in Texas; I can keep up with the latest news on the big sale of the Dallas Cowboys, my favorite NFL football team of all time. The news has kept me in an uproar for days. That's probably why I'm still sitting here at 5:30 A.M.; I was too upset to sleep last night.

I am in a state of shock! Like every red-blooded dyed-in-the-wool, true-blue (and silver) Dallas Cowboy fan, I'm furious that some Arkansas redneck named Jerry Jones has used his oil money to take over America's team. My heart bleeds for Tex Shram, and my tears flow for Tom Landry.

I may be from Louisiana, but I know every Texan believes this man ranks third in their life, only behind God and Mother. (Some folks don't even put them in that order!) He's somewhere in my top ten list, for sure, but I won't name names or ranks.

With a sports addict son like Billy, I was proud when he was growing up that there were men like Tom Landry for him to admire and respect. It isn't often you find a man with the integrity, honesty, and Christian leadership this man displayed, on and off the field. The only word to use as a definition is CLASS. (He had it; he showed it.) Jerry Jones and Jimmy Johnson can't buy that, or take it away from him.

What a shame it is that Mr. Jones paid $140 million dollars for the Dallas Cowboy franchise, and then tossed aside the only thing that made it worth that high price. It is truly a day of mourning for all Cowboy fans when this black shadow of shame has been cast on the Cowboy star, both the man and the emblem. Landry's firing and the way it was handled is probably an indication of what the future will bring: Victory above all, at all cost.

I know, I know, but why can't we have it all???? There are so few great heroes left in this world. Would it have been so hard for Jones and Johnson to have done the right thing? Tom Landry should have been cheered, honored, paraded, and given a gold watch. He should have exited Texas Stadium with confetti falling on his gray felt hat as he waved farewell to the adoring fans.

There's a big difference in being kissed goodbye, and in being kissed off!

3/1/93

This was written years ago, and now the Cowboys are the Super Bowl Champs, the best team in the world, but in my heart I still carry this grudge because the term "winner" doesn't seem to fit my description of either Jones or Johnson.

One Hundred Fifteen

Weird Week's Travels

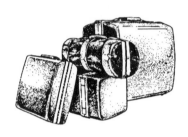

It has been a strange week for me on the road. I spent three nights in three different cities in three different hotels—all with poor tv reception. I did manage to watch the new Pat Sajak Show. I kind of like the show, but I feel guilty for not watching Johnny. I feel as if I'm cheating on him. We go back a lot of years. He's been a dear and faithful friend since my high school days; I can't leave him for a young upstart from Wheel of Fortune.

Anyway, enough about Johnny and Pat. I want to talk about people on airplanes. Do you ever wonder why they're there and where they're going? I like to try to match people to their occupations. Because I take a lot of Friday afternoon flights, I see many girls flying to meet guys and vice versa. That always results in a lot of kissing and carrying on in the airport. If you ever want to kiss, hug, and God knows what else without any one caring, go to the airport. You don't have to catch a flight, just hang around and make out. Everyone else does.

When people look tired and drawn, I figure they're headed home after a hard week on the road. If they cry a little, I assume there's been a death and they're flying home for the funeral... unless it's a Las Vegas outbound flight, then I know they're just mourning their losses and empty pockets.

Returning cruisers are the worst. They're red and parched and still ridiculously dressed in floral shirts and white shorts, even if it's 30 degrees in their destination city. They're loaded down with tax free whiskey, big straw baskets, and wide brim hats that say Bahamas. (Ever wonder how long before those hit the dumpster?)

Traveling from Houston to Dallas or the other way around on the Friday afternoon route is a disaster. It's filled with young travelers, some almost babies, making that weekend trek to visit their divorced Dad or Mom, as the case may be. Then late on Sunday, the same scene is repeated in the opposite direction. Both flights can be a travelers nightmare, but I feel more for the children than the flight attendants and fellow passengers.

I recently read that by the year 2000, a child without two sets of parents will be the oddball. Everyone will have at least two mommies and two daddies, not to mention how many uncles. I tend to agree with Roseanne Barr, "Why can't these people just hang in there and fight it out!"

Kids do not need frequent flier mileage!

One Hundred Seventeen

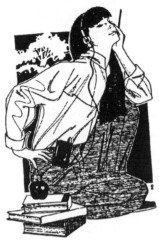

Missing Laura Lea

The empty nest syndrome would not get to me; I promised. I am a woman of the baby boomer generation. My life has meaning; it has purpose. Children leaving home will just mean more time for me; opportunity to pursue my career and personal development... NOT!

I hadn't realized how much I missed her until last Sunday. That was the longest day of my life. I kept going upstairs into her room and straightening up everything that was already straight. The plaques were on the wall; the prom pictures were framed by the bed; the cheerleader pom-poms were stacked in a basket in the corner; the corsages, the fliers, the posters, the ribbons, everything... all in place.

Remember the old rock 'n roll song, "School is Out For Summer?" This year it has a true meaning to me, as I can't wait for my baby to come home. (Letting her go away to private boarding school for a semester sounded good in the beginning, but I am miserable.) I want to grab her and hug her and never let her go. (At least for a day or so!)

Peace and quiet are nice at times, but I long to trip over dirty towels on the floor, find half-empty Coke cans scattered around, hear the constant ringing of a phone, and be on foot because my car is at the beach. (I won't even complain about the floorboards filled with sand or the wet car seats.) All of these inconveniences seem like heaven to me at this moment, and I'm longing to experience them all again.

Today I've been thinking about a quote a friend sent me recently. Doesn't really have anything to do with Laura Lea, but perhaps plays an important role in where I am at this time in my life. I appear to be mellowing.

It reads: "I don't know what it's like to be old... but I think, it's living long enough to make a joke of the things that were once breaking your heart."

Today I'm 44!

It has been a wonderful birthday so far. Last night Larry and I went to Opelousas and joined my good friend, Sue for the Alabama concert. They are one of my favorite country music groups, and I thoroughly enjoyed the entire fun-filled evening.

At first, I wondered why Larry had been so easy to convince to go, but then I learned there was a BASS fishing tournament scheduled for today, so he's off somewhere on a river, celebrating my birthday, while I'm here at home playing with the typewriter. It really didn't matter because I got loads of cards from friends, and silly gifts, and a devilishly delicious cake from Miss Emma. It was made of whipped cream, coconut, and lots of other heavenly and fattening things I'll be sorry for next week. Tomorrow I get to do this entire birthday deal again as we go to Mother's house for another party-time. I'll probably gain at least ten pounds just in time for my most important fall fashion market in Dallas. I hope tent dresses are back in style; I think I'm gonna need one.

Today (May 20) is not only my birthday but the birthday of Cher Bono. You know the tall pretty half of the once Sonny and Cher? I've always tried to associate myself with her, feeling we were sort of sisters of the zodiac, so to speak. Four years ago something funny happened in our relationship. When I turned 40; Cher turned 39—again! Each year since then, she's been one year younger than me. Today's newspapers read, "Cher is 43!" I don't know exactly how this works, but I'm definitely paying very close attention to make sure she doesn't lose any more years before we're fifty!

This month's *Redbook* has a perfect article for me and all those other Baby Boomers who are hitting their 40's. It's an interesting and inspirational letter called, "Forty-something." It was written from one friend to another marking her 40th birthday. Needless to say, every word hit home with me.

I wholeheartedly agree with the writer that it is the best of all decades in my life. It's a time of self-knowledge, self-confidence, and above all, self-acceptance. It is a time of believing in one's own abilities and daring to venture forth. Yet it's a time of realizing if we fall in the venture, it's no big deal. We've all learned to deal with things we can't alter, have patience to overlook the petty things in life that once may have upset or even obsessed us. More than any other time in our life, it is a decade of SELF, a time when the children are older and responsible for themselves, and our parents are still healthy and independent.

It's an age of realizing not only do we not look like a movie star, there's no chance we'll ever be one. No knight in shining armor is coming; no talent scout will discover us; no lottery ticket for life will be drawn. What we see is what we get, and perhaps realizing and accepting that is our biggest step toward maturity and happiness.

I certainly do not mean forsake hopes and dreams, just understand they are dreams. There are new words we discover with age, such as decaffeinated, bran fiber, Retin A, and hormones. I'm beginning to experience "my own private summer," even in the dead of winter. A full length mirror confirms that it is all still there, just an inch or so lower than it used to be. Hope of losing ten pounds before summer for the bikini season is no longer an option; I'll just buy a one piece and a long cover-up!

One Hundred Twenty-One

Judith Viort's book, *WHEN DID I STOP BEING 20?* clearly defines this as a decade of mixed emotions, a time of acceptance, understanding, forgiveness, and sorrow. We discover we are no longer somebody's little girl (my mother might argue that point), but worst of all... we learn we are not immortal. People younger than us are dying, and no one is whispering softly, "But she was so young."

I remember at 16 I drove fast with no regard to accident or danger. Now at 44, I fasten my seat belt and pray no fool runs over me. My knees tell me when it's going to rain and my feet let me know when I've had a hard days work. My frosted hair is natural and I spend much more money on creams and lotions than I do on perfume.

At thirty, thirty-five, and forty, I wrote similar letters to myself and hid them away in the lockbox, hoping I'd be the one who'd get to read them at a later date. Today's letter will be put in the same spot. It said, "This is the best time of my life. I don't recall a happier time and would not go back in time for anything or anyone... oh, I don't know... maybe Tom Cruise... no, probably not, but can I leave my options open, in case he asks?"

I'm finishing this letter alone in our living room. Larry is off fishing, Laura Lea is away at school, and Billy just called from Los Angeles to say Happy Birthday. As I sit in the darkness, tears stream down my cheeks, not for me, but because on this happiest day in my life, a warm, funny, wonderful girl has lost a long hard-fought battle with a cancer that consumed, and today finally, conquered her body. At forty-three, Gilda Radner is dead. Oh God, she was so very young.

One Hundred Twenty-Two

Another Chapter of Life

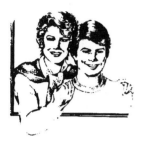

It's early morning as Delta and I take off headed to California. The airline breakfast was almost tasty; the weather is great; the blue skies up here are so beautiful I feel I must be in the palm of God's hand. Perhaps I am filled with expectation over my upcoming Los Angeles seminar or excited over spending a few precious days with my son, Billy.

I guess he's Billy today. Sometimes he decides to be Bill, on other days he likes William. I'm not always sure who to ask for when his secretary comes on the line, but I just love it when she says, "Can I tell him who's calling?" I embarrass him by saying, "His Mama," in my deepest southern drawl.

It's truly a strange feeling to see your child as an adult in their own environment. It's hard to comprehend they are no longer a resident in that "home" family, no longer a dependent on your income tax form, no longer your little boy. The realization of that moment brings mixed emotions of pride, joy, sorrow, and even perhaps envy.

For a few brief seconds, I think how exciting it would be to have a clean page on which to write my life story. What if hopes and dreams had a second chance to materialize, and choices had a second opportunity to be made?

Just as the bumper sticker reads, *"Grandchildren are God's gift of a second chance at parenting,"* I guess our own children are our second chapter to life's story.

Write on, Billy.

One Hundred Twenty-Three

Steel Magnolias and Weddings

Sherry got married this week. (You know, Billy's childhood sweetheart?) I cried throughout the entire ceremony. Even though she wasn't marrying Billy, it suddenly hit me, it could've been him. My days are probably numbered; I'm sure I'll be a mother-in-law in the next couple of years or so. Ouch... that has such a horrible ring to it. Even though I adore my mother-in-law, I seldom find anyone who has anything nice to say about theirs. Wonder what my daughter-in-law will be like? I'm sure as every mother says, "She certainly won't be good enough for him!" (Now that's probably why girls DON'T like their mothers-in-law, right?)

About Sherry's wedding... she was a beautiful bride, it was gorgeous, almost reminded me of the new movie, "Steel Magnolias." Go see it, you'll love it! It's the touching story of these strong Louisiana ladies and the trials and troubles they go through in life. The bridal preparations are the funniest scenes in the movie. Isn't the wedding usually the best part of the marriage? (Just kidding, Larry!)

The segments in Dolly Parton's beauty shop were more amusing in the play than the actual movie, although most of the dialogue has been left in tact. Robert Harling was hired to do the screenplay of his original work, and he gets to play a role in the movie. He portrays the preacher and does quite well for a non-professional actor, I think. It's good to see a Louisiana boy in the limelight! My favorite line from this sweet syrup version of Southern life is when Dolly says, *"The last romantic thing my husband did for me was enclose this here carport into a beauty shop, so I could make him a living."* Priceless, just priceless!

Don't listen to those Yankee movie reviewers on national television who are badmouthing this movie. So what if they showed a bayou scene in North Louisiana (they just got their geography a little mixed up!) What if they did the polka at a Cajun wedding in North Louisiana (I can forgive a musical mistake like that!). All minor faux paus. I didn't like them calling "ice tea, the house wine of the South" —that was tacky, but still, go see it! You'll laugh; you'll cry; you'll remember your grandmother, your mother, your daughter, your sister, your next door neighbor, and you'll realize just how much you love them and respect 'em all!

Welcome to the 90's

As we enter into the nineties, it is said we bid farewell to the decade of greed, and welcome the kinder, gentler era of George Bush's new America. In fashion and television, it's goodbye to Joan Collins and hello to Murphy Brown.

I started the year off right with the traditional New Year's Day dinner of cabbage, black-eyed peas, roast pork, etc. My best friend, Betty made me put a dime under my plate for luck (the first time I ever heard of that one, but I went along with it anyway), She better come through on her "get rich and stay healthy" guarantee. I'm counting on a great year ahead!

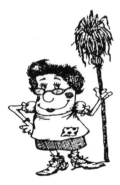

New Year's Day was a clean sweep time for me. I got a word processor from Santa Claus (ain't he sweet?), but didn't have anywhere to put it, so I decided January 1st was the perfect time to begin throwing away all the things I haven't needed or used in years. Unfortunately, cleaning came in a distant second to the trip down memory lane.

Everything I touched brought back some fond recollection from days gone by. I mean, who could throw away fifteen perfectly good Glen Campbell albums? Not me! Remember Larry and I saw him in concert on our very first date in 1968. Of course, I don't even own a record player anymore—everything is cassette and C.D., but Glen is staying! Same thing goes for the Peter, Paul, and Mary records, and Johnny Mathis, and the Kingston Trio. That's part of my history, right?

After nine hours of sorting through history (is the feminine of that called *herstory?*), I'm not any closer to finding a spot for the word processor. Maybe I'll just build a new office. That makes more sense to me rather than throwing away perfectly good stuff that I might need one day.

One Hundred Twenty-Seven

SUPER SUNDAY

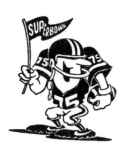

Boring? Dull? Worse game in Sunday Bowl history? Are you crazy? It was w-o-n-d-e-r-f-u-l; it was fabulous; it was one of the top ten experiences of my lifetime (I'll never name other dates or places, except for the 1982 State Basketball finals watching Billy make the All-State and the All-Star team). The other you'll have to guess or wonder about.

Perhaps the game was a bit one-sided, San Francisco 55—Denver 10, but I felt like Joe Montanas' Mama. Every time he broke a new NFL record, I cheered and yelled my heart out. Our seats were in the second level so we had a great eye view of everything. Even the poor Denver fans finally thought it was funny. What else could they do? (Before kickoff they were a bit happier and more cockier, but as all the buttons said, "JOE KNOWS FOOTBALL!")

From what I am told, the half-time show was a spectacular event with great costumes and grand performances from Irma Thomas and Pete Fountain. I can honesty say (cross my heart), I never saw a single one of them. When Laura Lea stepped on that stage, I saw her and her alone for the entire twelve minutes. My eyes never left her, even as she raced to the sidelines for costume changes. I watched her every moment, wanting to yell out to the crowds, "That's my baby!"

The tears streamed down my face from the beginning to the end; (people thought I must be a Denver fan with a big bet in Vegas). My heart pounded in my chest as I saw

One Hundred Twenty-Eight

her smile from the joy and excitement of participating in such a moment. I could see the tears rolling down her cheeks during the final numbers as the crowds cheered for more. Through soaking wet binocular lens I shared with her the emotional thrill of a lifetime.

All her griping about the hundreds of hours of practice and the daily drives to New Orleans for practice was suddenly wiped away by twelve minutes in the spotlight of the Superdome. Even though there were 50 All-American dance team members dressed exactly alike, and 500 additional dancers, and a total of 1800 people on the field at half-time, I only saw ONE, and one alone. For me, and Mrs. Montana, the Super Bowl 1990 is a Sunday we'll never forget!

February 14, 1990

HAPPY VALENTINE'S DAY, My Friend

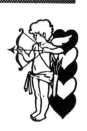

I rushed over to Modern Office Supply this afternoon, but I was just a little too late; Jeff had already closed. Yesterday when I went in there he and I got to talking about holidays and I completely forgot to buy Betty a card. I was so amazed when Jeff told me that Valentine's is his biggest card selling season, even more profitable than Christmas. It's always been my favorite holiday, but then I thought I was just one of those odd romantic hearts-and-flowers sort of people. I was glad to learn everybody else felt the same way. Still, this conversation made me forget Betty's card, and she's too important to me not to be remembered on February 14th.

Tonight I've found a verse in a book about friendship that I think I'll type and give to her tomorrow. Since I didn't see her tonight, I could just buy the card and she'd never even know I had purchased it a day late, but I like this message. I'm just gonna give her this, because it says all the things I want her to know.

"A friend is one with whom you dare to be yourself, a person who is not required to like you, but does, one who combines the pleasures and benefits of society and solitude, one soul in two bodies, someone you choose to be with. A friend is really a lot of things, a listener, a laugher, someone who says 'remember when we' and you remember. Friends finish sentences because that's the stuff friendships are made of. Sharing memories is the glue, and time polishes all real friendships until they shine."

I don't know who wrote this, but for now, it's me. Betty will understand.

One Hundred Thirty

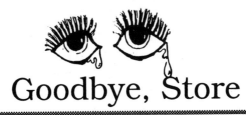

Goodbye, Store

This is a bittersweet day in my life, as I can't decide if I am happy or sad about deciding to close the store. It's such a difficult decision to give up twenty years of hard work, but it would be worse if I stayed.

My grandmother used to say, "A Jane of all trades is a master of none." Well, actually she said JACK, but she never heard of the E.R.A. or the women's movement. Lately this phrase has haunted me as I've tried to run the store, be a wife, raise a child, write a book, and travel all over presenting lectures and seminars. It just can't be done by one person; at least not done right.

Three weeks ago I looked into the mirror and remembered that line from "Steel Magnolias," *"Time is marching on, honey, right across your face!"* I could no longer pretend to be Superwoman, Erma Bombeck, Cher, Stanley Marcus, and Holly Homemaker—all rolled into one. There's just not enough of me to go around, and even though Cher and I share the same birthday, I can't sing.

The decision to close was easy after discussing it with my family. I felt a tremendous sigh of relief when Larry said, "Go for it!" He's always the wind beneath my wings that keeps me flying high. My sweet Renaissance girl child, Laura Lea delighted, "Wonderful, you deserve to rest, relax, and enjoy life." My ambitious California Yuppie son Billy's reaction, "Wow, now you can become rich and famous!" Three people, all related to me, all entirely different

One Hundred Thirty-One

reactions, opinions, and feelings, but they each shared and supported my decision in their own way.

Last year when I first began to ponder this change in my life, Margaret Gilley, a telephone friend, (we've never actually met in person but have spent hours chatting), sent me a quote which read, "*We must give up what we are for what we can become.*" It seems quite appropriate now as I leave one safe stage of my life and head off to try my hand at writing, speaking, whatever.

It's scary and certainly iffy, at best, but another quote I keep nearby says, "*You can't steal home plate with your foot on second base.*" I've made my choice, I'm already off and running towards third base. I just hope there is time enough in life to finish this home run!

The Academy Awards

What's it like to go to the Academy Awards? FANTASTIC, of course! I felt like Dorothy in the Wizard of Oz, except I came from Louisiana—not Kansas, and I wasn't wearing red shoes.

I spent most of the flight to L. A. convinced Delta would lose my luggage; then I worried that the flight would be late; then I decided Billy might just be joking about the whole thing. But no, it was a dream come true. Can you imagine a good looking young guy taking his mother to the Academy Awards? Well in 1990, two of them did. Billy Burch and Tom Cruise had some mighty proud dates that night. (By the way, I was with Billy!)

According to USA TODAY, "The hot ticket in town was the El Recate party, hosted by Reebok International," and yes, I was there! I was rubbing elbows with Dudley Moore, Jackson Browne, Jane Fonda, Robert Downey, Jr., Sally Kirkland, Daryl Hannah, Ted Turner, and all the other big stars. My only disappointment of the evening was when I was in the ladies room with Paula Abdul, Rob Lowe breezed through the bar and left. I missed that thrill!

There are no words to describe the experience and how I felt being there. After a while these people don't seem so great in real life. Jane Fonda actually looked old and wrinkled, but she has a great body. Dudley Moore was really short, and Daryl Hannah created a new word for tacky. Not only did she have on the ugliest dress I've ever laid eyes on, her hair looked like fried straw.

The food, the glamour, the decorations, even the ice sculpture that said REEBOK, were all too much for this country girl to believe. This fantasy land night will last in my memory forever... not so much because it was such a special event, but because my son chose me to share this evening with him. (Honestly, I think he looked a little bit better than Tom, but I didn't tell Mrs. Cruise that.)

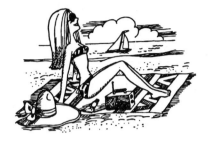

APRIL AT THE BEACH

If *"a rose by any other name is still a rose,"* then would Gulf Shores at any time, still mean SUMMER?

Last Friday everybody at my house (Larry, LaLea, and I) felt yucky. I was exhausted from traveling; Larry was tired of dealing with insurance; Laura Lea claimed homework overload. Actually the entire family was in an I.R.S. culture shock which didn't do much for our spirits or our bank account. Fortunately, instead of sitting around crying, we just decided to run away.

It took three toll-free calls, but a vacancy was located and in less than fifteen minutes from the first mention of the idea, the three of us were beach bound. Oh sure, we forgot a bunch of stuff, like clothes, toothbrushes, our usual load of rods, reels, and kites, but the thrill of just up and going without a moment's notice was fantastic. It was so out-of-character for me who knows where I'll be on November 12, 1991, and WHAT I'll be wearing.

It was a great weekend for the beach! I didn't dare put my toes in that icy water, but LaLea (that's her new abbreviated nickname) dove right in and shivered right out. Larry and I just sat on the sand, enjoyed the warmth of the sun, and took some leisurely strolls on the beach. It

One Hundred Thirty-Five

is times like these that make me think, modern medicine only invented VALIUM for people who can't go to the beach. The sounds of the waves and the smell of the ocean air would definitely cure me of almost anything that wasn't terminal or fattening.

Before heading home we stopped at Souvenir City; it's been a family tradition from the sixties. The place hasn't changed much. The walls are still bright neon colors, and decorated with hanging nets and shells and fish and ships and God knows what else. I did notice they had added a huge shark's head at the entrance which made for a real welcome sign!

While waiting for LaLea to finally make up her mind between two equally obnoxious teeshirts, I became interested in a conversation between two men, thirtyish, nice looking guys with a definite Yankee accent. One said, "I've been all over the world, but this place has to be the worst. I believe this is all the tacky in the whole entire universe rolled into one. God, this is horrible!"

Immediately, my feathers were ruffled. I walked over to them and put on my dumbest, deepest, southern accent and drawled, "Honey you ain't never been to Gulf Shores before, have ya?" I looked him up and down, and continued, "This here is heaven. My family's been coming here for over twenty years. We consider this almost a religious experience." (I gave him a lot to tell his New York friends when he returns home.)

Larry started laughing when we got in the car, and reminded me that it was the MOST tacky he'd ever seen in one place, and I had to agree with him, but it was OUR tacky place. That New Yorker had inspired in me a "love it or leave it" attitude about my favorite home away from home.

Returning to the beach at Gulf Shores every year is a renewal, a haven, a relaxing resting place where all is right with the world. The trials and troubles of every day life get washed away by the waves. The gritty sand between your toes, the bright neon bikinis, the loud pickup trucks, and the airbrushed teeshirts all mean the happy lazy days of summer... even on April 15th!

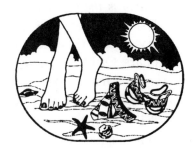

DIET or DENY IT?

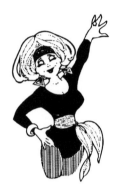

"*Today is the first day of the rest of your life*," another one of those stupid cheery quotes they throw at you in diet seminars. Or I really hate this one, "*Today is the tomorrow you planned for, yesterday.*" (Yes, when I was eating that banana split, I was thinking about tomorrow!)

Well, I'll take it seriously one more time. There has to be a way, right? Today I've weighed and measured, and I'm ready to see what happens. I want to have faith that I can do it.

Remember when I opened the store how fashionable I became? Then I opened the sunbed salon and became so very tan. Now, I've opened a Slenderizer Salon, shouldn't I become slim and trim? I'm working on it, but these machines aren't as user friendly as they promised. I don't want to do 524 simulated sit-ups in 10 minutes. (I feel very simulatedly sore after only two days!)

July 10. 1990

Nice try! My biggest problem is that I'm not the only enterprising business woman in my neighborhood this summer. Linda Binder has opened a snowball stand, just two doors down. A spearmint snow cone, topped with vanilla cream is a perfect picker-upper after a workout! (As a matter of fact, it's the best part of the workout.)

I've decided to rethink this situation. Summer is more than half over anyway; why worry about a swimsuit now? No diet; just deny it! I'm gonna ban the following words from the English language: flabby, dowdy, spread, middle

One Hundred Thirty-Eight

age, and over-the-hill. Attitude is everything. I can make up those catchy little phrases, too. Let's see...Um, "*Make the most of today, eat, drink, and move on to a happier tomorrow.*"

Just don't step on the scales. Works for me!

THE SEXIEST MAN ALIVE—1990

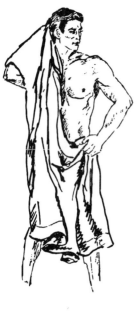

Yes, that's what the headline said. *People* magazine has selected TOM CRUISE as the sexiest man alive in 1990! So, didn't everyone already realize that? It was quite obvious the first time he danced across the screen wearing nothing but his jockeys and guitar! The writer said he was the star who can make a hit by just showing up. I bet that was a slur about COCKTAIL or DAYS OF THUNDER. Personally, I liked both of those movies; he took his shirt off several times, and did some great kissing scenes. Oh, certainly neither was another TOP GUN, but I'm not sure this old heart could take too many of those fantastic moments. Renting it once a month got so expensive, I finally just bought the video.

"He's Hollywood's sure thing with a killer grin and eyes to sigh for, at 5'7" he's a power packed hunk of heaven, at 28 years old"...how old, did they say? No, that's not right. My son is that age. There must be a typo here; they've made a mistake, I'm sure. Now you can't even believe what you read in PEOPLE!

August 1, 1990

DEAD POETS SOCIETY

Robin Williams was superb in the new movie, "Dead Poet's Society," but being an adult in the real world for longer than I'd care to admit, I couldn't get caught up in the excitement of the message. I vaguely remember those kind of days at Millsaps College. (We were all so very idealistic then; the campus was filled with ultra liberal intellects sporting beards, spouting poetry, majoring in the arts, and dreaming of renting lofts in Soho.) I recall wearing black turtleneck sweaters and pale white makeup, and typing sonnets by the light of a candle, melted repeatedly over the top of that very special wine bottle.

"Dead Poets Society" rekindled memories of those bittersweet days, but only for a few fleeting seconds. The most important thing this movie did was let me see the glow of idealism in Laura Lea's eyes as it's influence brought tears streaming down her cheeks. She returned to see the movie three times; each time viewing it through new inquisitive eyes looking toward the future. Oh, how I wish I could see life through the eyes of the young, but with the experience and wisdom of age.

My friend, Sue saw the movie this week also, and sent me this poem:

An 82 Year Old Looks Back

"If I had my life to live over, I'd try to make more mistakes next time. I would relax. I would limber up. I would be crazier than I've been this trip. I know few things I'd take seriously. I'd certainly be less hygienic. I'd take more chances. I would take more trips. I would scale more mountains. I would swim more

rivers. I would watch more sunsets. I would eat more ice cream. I would have more actual troubles, and less imaginary ones.

"You see, I was one of those people who would live sensibly and plainly by the hour after hour, day after day. Oh, I've had my moments, and if I had it to do over, I'd have more of them. In fact, I'd try not to have anything else, just moments, one after another, instead of living so many years on the safe side.

"I've been one of those people who never went anywhere without a raincoat and a parachute. If I had it to do all over again, I'd travel much lighter this time.

"I would start barefoot earlier in the spring, and I'd stay that way later in the fall. I would ride more merry-go-rounds, and dance more often. I'd catch more gold rings, greet more people, and pick more flowers ...if I had it to do over again, but you see I don't."

Second chances like those only come in movies. Remember Warren Beatty in "Heaven Can Wait?" Now, that was a movie!

One Hundred Forty-Two

What To Wear On QVC?

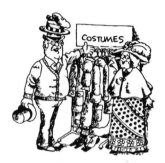

What does one wear for the most important event in their life? (No, I'm not getting married AGAIN, and for the other two most meaningful events of my life, the hospitals made me wear those ugly green gowns!) I'm talking serious event here; I'm talking national television debut on QVC next week, and I'm about to go crazy. Probably I'm just scared, but this wardrobe thing has become an obsession. (Not like Calvin Klein's Obsession—in my nightmares I have on clothes!)

For the past two weeks I've been in and out of every dress shop and department store within 200 miles of here. I think I've brought something home on approval from every store. (Don't you know they're just loving writing up those return credit slips?)

It has been a good lesson in customer service, though, and I'll probably be able to charge all this travel off my taxes as research for future marketing seminars. (Think the I.R.S. will agree?) Anyway, back to service—or lack of.

Saks Fifth Avenue in New Orleans has to get the worst score and as a matter of fact, I told them so in person and by letter. Even though my friend, Betty and I were the only two people in the entire department, we still couldn't get attention. When we finally did beg this harsh looking gray haired lady to wait on us, she was so rude she made us regret ever asking.

At Macys, it was the exact opposite; we were treated like royalty (crowns omitted). Betty casually lounged comfortably in a big overstuffed chair while the sales assistant zipped and buttoned and ran all over the place trying to find me the "perfect" outfit. When I saw the price tags, I knew why. I said, "Thank you, I'll come back when I decide," and then under my breath added, "and after I win the lottery."

Still, it's this week and what I am I wearing? Who knows! There's this really classy two piece crepe suit that makes me look like Susan Dey without the blonde hair and L.A. Law degree. Then there's a double-breasted coat dress that makes me resemble a white Oprah, less a few lumps and bumps. One form-fitting leather look was interesting, but I felt like an old Cher with thirty extra pounds and no tatoo.

If I wear a bow blouse, I'll feel dowdy and old; if I go with a low cut number I'll feel cheap and trashy. Red gives too many color shadows and turns orange on camera, but white is too bright and reflects off the lens. Black appears harsh and hard and brings out the wrinkles, and God, how I hate pastels.

Do I want to look warm and friendly or sophisticated and worldly? Should I be authoritative or passive and mild? If I don't smile, I'll look tense, yet if I grin, my crows feet will scrunch up. My right side is definitely the best, but if I turn my face too far around then my chin looks droopy. And what about the accent? Will they be able to understand me or will I just sound country? I can hear the producers now, "She's not a Southern Belle; she's a Southern Boob!"

One Hundred Forty-Four

Me who never sleeps at night, now can't even sleep in the day time. I'm up twenty-four hours a day worrying about this. I figure at this rate, I'll probably collapse from lack of sleep and miss the entire t.v. show anyway.

Seriously, I've decided to go to the closet (my own) and just find something to put on, one of my usual outfits. After all,these QVC folks didn't invite Susan Dey, Oprah, or Cher, so I guess I shouldn't surprise them by showing up as someone else. What's the quote? "Be yourself... No one else is better qualified!"

U.S. at WAR
Desert Storm Attack

While most people seem to have etched in their memories their exact location when they heard Kennedy had been shot, I for one, do not.

I don't know why I can't remember, it just seemed like IT HAPPENED, and everything before, right after, and during that period is still a blur.

Not so, that cold January 1991 day when Desert Storm began. I think I'll always remember every little detail, every thought, every feeling, every sound.

Larry and I had just completed a visit to QVC in Pennsylvania which included a side trip to Valley Forge and the Amish country. That Sunday morning we actually stood in Independence Hall and sensed the presence of Ben Franklin standing proud there in debate. John Hancock's pen still lays across the papers on the scroll top desk where he so boldly scribbled his name, and we saw the house where young Betsy Ross spent long hours sewing together colorful bits of fabric into stars and stripes. Even now at this moment my hand can still feel the coolness from the metal of the Liberty Bell where my fingers traced over the famous crack. We had felt the pride of our heritage and learned more of the history of our ancestors and our country.

At Valley Forge we viewed the Army bunkers and read monuments and tributes to our early war heroes. What pride and sorrow we felt for those 2,000 young men who died that terrible winter, not from war but from the bitter cold and disease, as they awaited the British army.

At 5:45 p.m. Larry and I landed home in New Orleans, where we first learned of the Desert Storm attack; we turned on the radio as we were leaving the airport parking lot. The initial shock brought tears and worry, but thankful prayers that we were home in safe surroundings with those we loved.

Abruptly—it was not Valley Forge. It was not 1776; it wasn't Tom Cruise in "Top Gun" or one of my uncle's old war stories. It was 1991 and the real thing!

Born in 1945, I was a child during Korea, and an indestructible naive teenager at the time of Vietnam. Today as a grown adult, I could truly comprehend and understand the terror of war, and I am scared. I have a past I cherish, a present I cling to, and a future I hope for. My world, yesterday so secure, today seems so fragile.

Do people ever grow old enough to understand war?

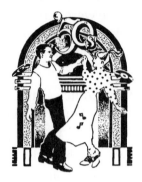

Is it Thee, Sandra Dee?

One of the reasons I enjoy visiting and working on the west coast is the time zone difference. My body is still adjusted to CST. I wake up at 6 A.M. in California. (My body thinks it's 8 A. M., so I have some extra time to write or watch early morning television, something I never get to do at home.)

Last week I was switching channels in Los Angeles, when I heard a familiar voice from the past. I stared almost in disbelief at the haggard, puffy, tired, bleached blonde stranger on the screen. Not until she said, "And when I first married Bobby Darin...," did I dare let myself believe this was SANDRA DEE? I was heart broken; I was devastated. To me, Sandra Dee was a young, petite, beautiful girl, frolicking on the beach wearing a polka dot bikini, holding hands with Tab Hunter, while strains of "A Summer Place" played in the background. (If you're too young to remember, Tab Hunter was the 60's version of a blonde Tom Cruise without acting ability!)

My California day went down hill from this and turned into a weekend of de ja vous. The Cal-Mart fashion shows were a visit to Back-to-the-Future (no Michael Fox). Everyone in the audience over age forty felt they were reliving Woodstock, Camelot, and Beach Blanket Bingo with Frankie and Annette. I sat there in shock as I watched my entire teenage wardrobe parade down the runway on models who looked like my best friends from Kentwood High School in 1962. I swear one of them had on my favorite purple bracelet she borrowed that spring, and never returned!

What's NEW in fashion? Nothing it's all recycled from the past. Those little flip dresses were shown in bursts of hot pink, lemon lime, purple, and orange. Covering the legs was a necessity because these little numbers barely covered the fanny, so leggings were shown in wild Pucci prints with open-toe slingback mules, circa 1960. Faces in the show were framed with bouffants from the Kennedy White House, Audrey Hepburn's famous beehive, and Mary Tyler Moore's glued-in-place flip do.

It seemed like a hoot, but the unfunny part was, these designers were serious. What goes around, comes around, and 1960 has returned. For those of us who wish to forget pimples, cheerleading, and the prom, our wardrobe choices will be limited to what's left over from last season, unless you follow my fashion advice:

Treat yourself to a new trendy look. It'll look great for that thirtieth class reunion this summer. Don't despair if your budget is tight. Just drop by your Mama's house and start digging through the upstairs closet. I bet somewhere behind the waterskis, the hula hoop, and the Elvis records, you'll discover stacks of 1991 designer creations.

Take 'em out, stand in front of the mirror, and try 'em on. If they still fit, you're in great shape. Give yourself a pat on the back, and smile as you say, "Eat your heart out, Sandra Dee!"

Happy, Wealthy, and Wise

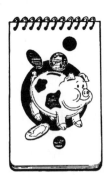

Today I read a quote, *"The days that make us happy, also make us wise."* If that is true, I must be the smartest lady around these days. My life has recently been a whirl wind of travel, writing, and speaking.

Laura Lea and I went to New York and experienced it to the fullest: Glamour, glitz, glory, and gore—all in one trip. We took in a couple of plays, went to the ballet, shopped all the high fashion stores, visited SoHo and the Village, and risked our lives (I am sure) touring the burned-out sections of the Bronx. Just our luck, we got to witness the police pulling a dead body from the East River, as well as a mugger stealing a lady's handbag outside the theater. Oh yes, New York and all it's fun. We were even in town for the Desert Storm Victory ticker-tape parade. (I've never seen so many people in red/white and blue in my entire life. The island of Manhattan looked like one big American flag!)

In addition to New York, I've been on the road lately to Dallas, Denver, Tampa—all over the place, but best of all—I've been home for awhile. It's been great fun, just playing house—no cooking involved. When I play house, I redecorate, and I'm redoing everything in black and white. Larry claims I'm dangerous with a spray can; he thinks if it stands still, I'll paint it!

Cat, beware !

One Hundred Fifty

My new dining room is my pride and joy. It's been over fifteen years since I changed it, so it was definitely time for an updated look. It's black and white, of course, with lots of stripes and dots, accented with cows. Yes, I said c-o-w-s. I even have the fabulous dishes from Saks Fifth Avenue and the silverware with the cow handles! (Please, don't moo; I hear enough of that from my family!)

The room wasn't completed a day too soon as it's been in constant use as our social center. First, I entertained the girls from Laura Lea's high school graduating class with a senior luncheon. (It's sort of a Southern thing, like a coming out party or a Sweet Sixteen Party, Mason-Dixon Mamas can't resist!) Then on graduation night, the family gathered to toast in celebration using the 150 year old wine glasses from Larry's grandmother's plantation home, Fairview. (The glasses have only been used once in 25 years—gives you some idea how happy we were over this graduation!)

Next, we rejoiced in another important event as Billy flew his California girl to New Orleans so he could propose to her in the Louisiana moonlight. The next day they and their friends filled our house and our dining room with joy as we showed them a thing or two about Cajun food and eating crawfish.

Only days later it was Mother's 65th birthday, and I decided she needed a surprise party. With help from her friends, I was able to pull it off and she didn't suspect a thing. The dining room was filled with cake, punch, birthday goodies, and good friends and family.

I'm really crazy about this room. Wonderful, happy, exciting things are happening there all the time lately....but, I just got on the scales. Now I'm not sure how much of this happiness stuff I can stand. I'm thinking of rewriting that philosopher's quote to read: "The days that makes us happy, also make us W-I-D-E!"

One Hundred Fifty-One

Steel Magnolias and Fried Chicken

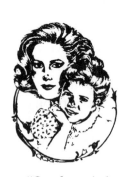

While traveling, I constantly buy books and magazines to read on the plane. This week in Houston's Hobby Airport I came across a book *Southern Is...* Of course, I had to buy it, just for the name, but I soon read it, and re-read it, and read it again.

The little book explains just what Southern is in such statements as: *"Southern is knowing where your people come from, how they got there, where they're buried, who married who or should've and didn't."* Boy, does that sound familiar. I had an Aunt Jessie who could tell the history of the Phillips family back to the Civil War. Unfortunately, she often did tell it, whether anyone wanted to hear it or not.

On those long afternoons, I spent as a child lying on the bed with my grandmother, I would listen to her stories of all the weird aunts or the outcast uncles or the distant cousins, some of which we liked, some of which we avoided, but all which we loved. Southern families always seem to have at least one strange distant relative who buried their money or ran away with a traveling salesman, or God forbid, married a Yankee and moved up North.

My grandmother was a hard working woman. She was up at three every morning getting ready to open the school cafeteria by four-fifteen A.M. sharp. Mrs. Beatty had to be there early to get those hot rolls rising and those chicken and dumplings cookin' for the children's lunch.

She was home by two p.m.; that's when she would lie down on her little cot and teach me how to read and write, or tell me stories from the past or make up tales about the future. Even though she was the best cook in this entire part of Louisiana, she never taught me a thing about the kitchen. I can still hear her saying over and over, "Honey, you're too smart to be cooking for anybody. You're gonna be somebody one day." (I often think of how proud she would be of my writing career, but I still wish I knew how to bake those wonderful cinnamon rolls.)

In that little book I bought, it said, "*Southern is fried chicken.*" Oh, how true this statement is, and the memories it brings back. A long list of preachers sat at my grandmother's table during her lifetime. At least one Sunday a month, usually two, some preacher and his family from somewhere or other were coming to call, and there were chickens to be killed and dumplings to be made. Although I never participated or even watched, I can still hear that eerie cackling sound of the main dish's demise. Plucking chicken feathers was almost fun sometimes, if ya hadn't been asked to do it. (The feathers were later dried and saved for making pillows, special pillows for special people.)

One of the best family traditions that began at my grandmother's house, and continues on today at my mother's, was "in-law food." Did you ever have that at your house? My mother puts the fried chicken on the platter, but saves the wings and the wishbone on a separate saucer. Larry and Laura Lea are dared to touch them—they're for me! Pies were my JoJo's in-law specialty. There was a certain lemon cheese (chess) pie for Mattie Lea (my mother), a coconut pie for Sugar (my aunt), and a lemon pie for my Uncle R.E. If a daughter-in-law or son-in-law happened to like the same variety of pie, that was fine, but no one was allowed to cut any pie until the chosen one arrived. As I said, there was

One Hundred Fifty-Three

family members pie, and there was in-law pie, the first of the two was always the best!

"Southern is knowing a woman who made a career out of being a lady." That was definitely Larry's grandmother, Miss Lucy. It was in early 1969 that she summoned me to afternoon tea in the big house (a huge three story turn-of-the-century structure that scared me on sight). She sat there so erect in her white blouse trimmed high at the neckline in lace, her navy linen skirt so starched and proper, and her beautiful gray hair swept up in bun. Tiny little wisps gracefully fell and framed her face, and she worn a single strand of pearls—real pearls. She served home-made cookies on antique dishes and coffee in dainty cups with heavy silver spoons (the weight of the real stuff), and told me the family history dating back to her plantation days. She loved to remember when Pops, her husband was Huey P. Long's attorney, and repeatedly told the tales of his shenanigins up and down the parish and throughout the entire state. Meme didn't think much of Mr. Long, but he was a regular houseguest at the Reid's for many years. When Larry and I married, Meme gave us "The Huey P. Long" bed as a wedding gift. It's a huge brass four poster we'll cherish forever. Pops had given it to her as a bride in 1912.

Meme (as the children called Miss Lucy) lived well into her nineties, but 'til the day she passed away, she rose every morning and got dressed up exactly the way she was the first day I met her. Never did she go without stockings, never did she forget that powder or just a little tinge of rouge, never was a hair out of place, and the pearls, she wore them to her grave. In the dictionary under lady, the definition is surely Miss Lucy.

"Southern is talking 'bout Jesus like he lived next door." I never really thought about that, but I guess Southerners do have a rather personal, familiar kind of relationship with the Lord. After six years of piano lessons (all 2,021

days my mother forced me to practice), to this day thirty-six years later, I can still only play two songs from memory. One is "What a Friend We Have in Jesus" and the other one is "Love Me Tender." Well, what can I say, we think Elvis lives here now, too!

Letters

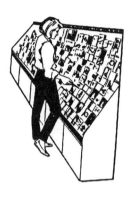

I've already confessed to you that I write letters to myself and hide them. I guess that sounds rather strange, especially from a woman my age, but I started this early in my childhood. Perhaps I should have called it a diary or journal, but really they were and are, actual LETTERS TO ME, things I want to think about, savor, enjoy, and try to understand.

In this fast paced world of television, computers, and faxes, too many people are overlooking the value of letters. Although I am a self-admitted phone-aholic, I've never lost my love for the written word. The rewards of long lasting hand scribbled notes can never be replaced or equalled by South Central Bell, MCI, or Sprint, no matter what Candice Bergen tells ya.

My favorite way to start the day is with the morning mail. It delights me even on the first of the month when the unpaid bills are stacked sky high. I have a system for opening my correspondence. First I look at all the junk mail—just a quick glance, filing the keepers and tossing the rest. After the trash mail, I look at the bills, then the business letters, then the fun begins!

I experience a sense of excitement when a colored envelope or a postcard stands out among the Publisher's Clearinghouse winner announcements. I feel a tingle of anticipation at the sight of a familiar handwriting or postal mark. Sometimes years may have passed but I can still

One Hundred Fifty-Six

recognize the beautiful script or the messy scrawl of a friend.

After savoring this initial moment, I tear into the envelopes and read very quickly to find out all the details and latest news. Then I sit back and delight in a second reading, every word read and reread two or three times to grasp the feelings. I enjoy attempting to read between the lines to sense what affection, anxiety, or happiness the writer may have intended.

Favorite letters or cards are among my most prized personal possessions. Usually greeting cards on any holiday are more important than the actual gifts they accompany. Unlike those romantic ladies of yesteryear, I do not tie them up in lace ribbons with pressed flowers, but I keep them pinned on bulletin boards or stuffed in desk drawers or packed away in shoe boxes. Occasionally. I'll take the time to reminisce through correspondence from months or even years ago, and experience again, the same warmth and closeness I felt the first day it arrived.

With both children away from home, our phone bill is tremendous. I love speaking to them regularly , but what I cherish most is their letters. Billy's are always short, quick memos, scribbled with great humor and sarcasm. He uses Reebok notepads or funny post-it notes, each and every single one signed, "Your Son, Billy." It's been a family joke for so long that Laura Lea does the same, "Your daughter, Laura Lea." (I assume they each want to clarify their identity and relationship to us, in case we have forgotten them during their absence.)

Billy's are funny, and always enjoyable, I laugh as I read them over and over. Laura Lea's letters are a breath of fresh air, and a day of sunshine. Her bright colorful stationery is adorned with funny faces and notes; she even covers the envelopes. I'm filled with joy before I get a chance to open each potential work of art. She makes little

One Hundred Fifty-Seven

sketches, changes ink colors for each word, creates "new" words, and literally pours her heart and soul out onto each page. I read her letters over and over, and each time they're unfolded, more love flows from the paper. (I can only imagine the pleasures I'll receive when reading these around the year 2020!)

Too many people today consider themselves too busy to write letters. What a waste! I have a friend, Donna, a delightful woman from Arkansas who once penned me a 32 page manuscript. It took her four hours to carefully word this saved-up friendship that she so beautifully shared with me. I was deeply touched, and it's one of my prized possessions. My cousin, Ramona has a talent for selecting cards that are right-on- target, and never fails to bring a smile to my face. My friend, Carroll is another person who always sends cards and notes when they are appreciated the most, but the majority of people just don't do that anymore.

Letters and cards are nourishment for the soul. They can be used to express words, too often unspoken, and feelings seldom communicated. They provide friendship, warmth, love, advice, and even at times—criticism, without the interruption on the other end of the line. Some need to be responded to, while others are simply filed away in my heart and memory (and shoe boxes).

My correspondence is either by funny cards—I love the Hallmark Shoebox cards (I secretly think I AM THAT LADY!), or on yellow legal pads written on airplanes or in hotel rooms late at night. If I feel "up," I can pour that energy into page after page of inner secrets to friends, loving advice to my children, or sometimes I write the history of the world today, as I see it. These outbursts are never regular or scheduled; I may write five in one night or one in a week, depending on my mental state. Though the words are meant for the reader, I am the one who receives a total, almost cleansing, sensation when the thoughts are transferred from my mind to the paper.

If you are reading this and can think of someone you need to write, STOP! Do it today. Take the time to share yourself with someone you care for. Skip WHEEL OF FORTUNE for 30 minutes, and use words not to fill in the blanks with Vanna White, but to relay meaningful messages. It requires so little of your time, and someday these letters may be part of a cherished collection of someone's life memories. They can definitely be part of their today's smile.

Ma Bell may claim to reach out and touch someone, but the pen is mightier than the phone. Words can be enjoyed many times over, long after the phone bills have been paid. I am so thankful for a mother who gave me the important things in life: roots, wings, and a BIC pen!

A New Year's Resolution

Be Nice to Yourself!

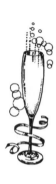

It's January 1st, but it's not just the first day of a new year, it's the start of your diet plan, isn't it? In less than two weeks, some of us will be soaking our aerobic-strained muscles, while others will be blending and shaking those chalky-tasting chocolate flavored liquids that Tommy LaSorta swears tastes, "Yummy!" Many will be weighing carefully and measuring each tiny morsel of veggies, while yet others will be rushing and running full-speed ahead from the exceleration of their new expensive diet wonder pills. Yes, they'll be making those extra bathroom stops so necessary now from the little fluid tablets the miracle doctor also prescribed. Some will choose to go it alone—brave the venture without support from others, while many will return to those special weight group meetings where they are forced to publicly weigh in, and describe their criminal eating habits to all in attendance.

"Are we having fun yet?" It's so sad, but true, each and every January 1st at least 50% of the entire population goes on a diet. Unfortunately in less than thirty days, 90% have already broken the New Year's Resolutions and gone back to normal daily lifestyle B.D. (Before Diet!)

A recent survey said 85% of all resolutions involved two topics: Weight and Wealth, or as I like to name them: Looks and Loot! I guess we just want to have it all. Lose

One Hundred Sixty

ten pounds, make more money, and get more goodies! That's the American dream that we plan for, hope for, and promise to achieve—each and every January 1st.

Two weeks from now, don't hate yourself or feel like a failure if all you've lost is your temper, your sense of humor, and fourteen days! Just look into the mirror and see deep down into the real person reflected there. Are you happy, content, complete, and fulfilled? Isn't that what really counts? Dwell on spending your time and energy doing the things you enjoy, being with the people you love, and learning to take control of your life.

The book, *On A Clear Day You Can See Forever* talks about all the wasted times in our lives. When we are young, the days never seem to pass fast enough. We dwell on the future, thinking, "When I grow up ...when I marry ...when I move away...," then so quickly it seems we are older and start to look back at the past, living in thoughts of "If only ...I wish I had..." and so our life stories go.

My New Years Wish for me and each of you is that in this coming year, we become the person we want to be—not in dreams, but in reality. I'm well past young and planning ahead, but I'm feeling far from the looking back stage. This is my time of the present—my NOW to enjoy and live each single day to its fullest. I'm sure LOOKS AND LOOT are nice, but they aren't even near the top of the list of hopes for the coming year. There are TOO many important things in life that really matter.

One Hundred Sixty-One

The Maine Event

My friend, Louise had promised to show me the entire Northeast, but I never expected her to be able to do it in twenty-four hours. The states are so small, it only took a couple of hours for us to go from Connecticut all the way to Maine. On arrival, I realized it was exactly what I had thought it would be: wet. (Ever wonder why it always rains in Maine? Maybe because it rhymes.) Anyway, folks were all running around in those little yellow slickers and the entire scene looked like something out of the script of *MURDER SHE WROTE*, minus Angela Landsbury.

I immediately headed for the high points and thoroughly enjoyed looking at the multi-million dollar homes on the way up the coast to Kennebunkport. I was surprised to find we were able to drive right up to Barb and George's house with no trouble at all. It's hard to miss with all the flags, the helicopter pad, and the G-Men hanging 'round. Still, they let us take photos and tour the immediate area (the folks were away), until some guy finally motioned us on. What an amazing discovery I made. If you've been wondering what happened to Ken Wohl from the WISEGUY television series; he's now in the Secret Service guarding George's place. (He's still quite a hunk—no Tom Cruise, but a hunk anyway!)

The actual town of Kennebunkport is a pure tourist delight. These folks are making a mint off everything from Presidential seals to Millie the Dog bath mats. There are blocks and blocks of nothing but gift shops all along the waterfront and a few good restaurants that advertise, what else, but clam chowder and lobster! Cash registers are ringing; money is trickling down; it's a Republican Paradise.

It was early July, and I was dressed in a teeshirt and shorts. The low 60's temperature combined with the drizzling rain were causing me to get the chills, so I set out to find warmer duds. Since I meant to buy a souvenir anyway, a sweatshirt seemed ideal.

Ideal, until I looked at the price tags!

There were Barbara shirts, Maine shirts, George shirts, Millie shirts, but certainly no c-h-e-a-p shirts. The most reasonable (ha) one I could locate said "SUMMER WHITE HOUSE," and it cost $39.95, on sale, marked down from $50.

Noticing my southern drawl, the owner came rushing over to close the sale on this nifty little item himself. "Can I help you with a shirt, missy?" he smiled his best Yankee after-my-money grin. "No, I don't believe so," I said. "I'm just cold and looking for something inexpensive to cover up with." He quickly responded, "Oh, you'll really enjoy this SUMMER WHITE HOUSE shirt. It'll last you all next winter, too."

That was the opportunity I couldn't let pass, so I turned on my best southern charm (the United Daughters of the Confederacy would've been proud!), and said, "Yes sir, it would, but by next winter the summer white house is gonna be in Little Rock, ain't it?"

With a little tenseness in his expression, he cleared his throat, kept those teeth shining and answered, "You're probably right, young lady, you're probably right."

He was a greedy Yankee Republican, the shirt was overpriced, but the man was smart—he'd called me YOUNG, plus he had the wisdom to know, the party was over. I immediately liked the fellow.

P.S. You ought to see my Kennebunkport sweatshirts. I got two of those dillies!

One Hundred Sixty-Three

3/1/93

(The Yankee and I were both right, by November Bill Clinton was president. Arkansas was in; Maine was out. Wonder what shirts are selling for in Hot Springs and Little Rock?)

I'm Voting for Hillary's Husband!

A s the election time draws near, it seems one of the most vital issues of the campaign has become the wive's wardrobes. Last week a national headline read: "Washington Woes: The Year of the Woman." Then the article proceeded to discuss, not childcare, not abortion issues, not equal pay, not even women running for office. It was strictly about what the candidate's wives were wearing. (Now is this a great country or what?)

I realize Barbara Bush has made a multi-millionaire out of Kenneth Jay Lane with those stupid three strand pearls of hers, "But enough already, Barb. We know you've got three chins; stop trying to hide them and just be the role model the plus size women want you to be." She adds such esteem and self-confidence to the fuller-figure ladies, but then turns around and says she wears a size 14-16. "Get real, Bar. You're a 1X if I ever saw one, honey. Admit it, no one cares. We all like chocolate chip cookies, too."

With Marilyn along, Barbara will always look terrific. Let's face facts, here. Marilyn has terrible taste in everything from hats to husbands. She needs to retire to the background and give Dan spelling lessons. (I think there'll be plenty of free time ahead for such family activities.)

It's hard to make a decision on Hillary's wardrobe or her image. It looks like she buys her stuff off-the-rack (a plus for us retailers), and we know she serves on the board of directors for Wal-Mart. (I don't think she's picked up any outfits there!) Ann Taylor, Casual Corner, Dillards, all look like Hillary's type apparel. Wouldn't it be great to have a First Lady who shopped where we did? (But will it last? Probably not. They'll force her to go the way of others before her, and she'll become a couture queen for designers like Valentino or Chanel.)

The headband has got to go, but I think it already has. Linda Bloodworth-Thomason has put the brakes on the hairdo by bringing in a Hollywood hairstylist to put a little bounce in that bob. So far so good on the Hillary fashion report; I'll keep a close eye for late breaking news; I'm sure it'll make the UPI before any important announcement of policy.

I can't tell much about Tipper. When she stands next to Al—who looks? (The man is a hunk; no Tom Cruise, but a hunk anyway!) I think Tipper's preppy no-nonsense look comes straight out of the J. Crew mail order catalog. I know it'd make any Ole Miss sorority sister jump with joy. Hopefully, if he's elected she'll donate her duds to some university, and graduate on up to adult dressing.

Think her taste in music has anything to do with her taste in clothing?

Are you reading this and laughing, or do you realize just how ridiculous this is? These are not serious factors to ponder when entering a voting booth. None of this trash on trends and fashion makes any sense at all to me when the Presidency of the United States is at stake. The future of our country, our children, our world is in our hands in November. Don't take this lightly!

Who should represent THE WOMAN OF THE NINE-TIES? Is it going to be a cookie baking grandma who

One Hundred Sixty-Six

writes about puppy dogs and walks two steps behind her master, George, or do you prefer the straight talking feminist who up front says, "You're getting both of us.?" There is no decision here for me; my choice is made. I don't want to turn back the hands of time; I want my daughter to step forward into a new century of equality, or at least a semi-shot at it.

Personally, I'm a sale shopper. I like the bargain offer that Hillary and Bill have made. I think it's time America and women got their money's worth. I'll take the two-for-one sale. Put it on my Visa, please!

GRUNGE in the 90's

"Happy Days are here again, the skies are..." That's the song we've been hearing out of Washington since the election, but the songs coming out of Seattle have had much more effect on our fashion culture than any presidential hoopla Bill could've started.

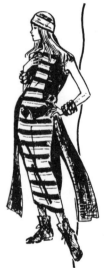

The word is called GRUNGE, a nickname given a bunch of semi-dirty, half-dressed rock musicians, who are gaining fame in the Northwest. This fashion trend, if it can be called that, is rather anti-fashion, promoting a "thrown together" messy, mismatched mood of style. These folks consider themselves well-dressed in fingerless gloves, midriff-baring crop tops, stocking caps, and anything that's too long, too short, too loose, or too tight! That's what GRUNGE is all about— being different, and loving it.

It's really nothing new, reminds me of the sixties. The dresses resemble somebody's grandma's living room curtains, and the stocking caps look like just that—stockings. There are even models walking around with their navels exposed above the belts of their bell bottom hip hugger pants, and bunches of daisies stuck in their hair.

Why now, Lord? Why did you bring this plague on America's retailers just when the economy looked like it might turn around? Why curse us with a season of no business? People only need to return to their Mama's attic or some old thrift shop to garner an entire spring 1993 wardrobe. Store owners need them at the cash registers with their wallets open.

Anyone over thirty-five has lived through this look before, and even liked it BACK THEN. I remember my extreme bad taste in 1971 when I wore a skinny ribbed teeshirt (it was bright purple), and donned a pair of pants with wide bold vertical stripes of purple, gold, tan, red, and green. (Please, try not to throw up over this color combination. I thought it was c-o-o-l, at the time.)

Last night I rummaged through old photo albums trying to find the picture of me in that gorgeous get-up. I remember having at least one or two memorable moments captured on film in that outfit. I searched for hours with no luck, so I finally decided at some time in the eighties I must have come to my fashion senses and destroyed the photographic evidence that I had ever worn such terrible clothing. (Smart move!)

Laura Lea has started wearing old love beads and peace symbols, so I may dig out some of my "hippie" leftovers for her. I guess it is sort of a return to the sixties. We have a new Kennedy-like president who has promised us a new Camelot, though I doubt Hillary wants to be Jackie O. We as American shoppers, have embraced the reverse snobbery and now brag about how little we pay for something, rather than how much. In 1988, who would've ever thought it could happen that way? People are driving 1988 model BMW's over to Sam's Wholesale Club, buying toilet tissue on sale, in bulk!

Grunge, sponge, whatever they call it, it's strange, but I guess it's fashion 1993 style. Like every other decade and it's fads, it'll catch on and I'll have to participate. My biggest worry at the moment: "Is America ready to see my belly button again?"

I think not.

One Hundred Sixty-Nine

Lauri, What Fun We Had!

I t is hard to type the words: Lauri passed away. Maybe I could just say, Lauri passed my way. What a wonderful way to think about her!

She was one of my first customers in the store when I opened. Of course she was a hard-to-please spoiled little teenager at the time, but who could get aggravated at Lauri? Well, everybody, but who could stay aggravated at Lauri? No one! Even then, her personality lit up a room when she entered.

I don't exactly recall when she stopped calling me "Miss Tommy Jean," and started with "T.J.," but as she got out of school and married, we became more than merchant and shopper. We were friends.

Both of us had a thing for crazy, silly, obnoxious cards, and would try to out do each other. Sometimes I'd search racks for hours to find just the right greeting for Lauri, and she'd still be one up on me.

Nobody ever loved clothes better than that girl. She was a walking advertisement for my store, every time she stepped out of the house, even if it was jeans and a sweatshirt. Lauri had a way of looking special! Earrings were her favorites; I think she owned a hundred pair, but still would buy more! It really hurt my business because women would say, "I'll just borrow some from Lauri. I know she's bound to have a pair to match my outfit!" (And she did; she could match every outfit in everyone's closet!)

Sometimes we would hide the monthly statement from Danny, but when she had him put up that rack that was supposed to hold eighty pair and had some left over, I think he knew!

When she first started her fight with the cancer, there was no doubt, she'd beat this thing. Cancer didn't know who it was messing with! She'd smile and make jokes about her new hair do, and show off her endless supply of wigs in all styles. Sometimes she'd laugh and share her Sinead O'Conner impression, and actually for a time make you believe, she really didn't hurt. She never gave in; she always believed she could make it.

Having her as a model in the video, ACCESSORY ADVANTAGE: TACKY To TERRIFIC was her idea. She wouldn't hear of letting me do this without her. Lauri was always a STAR! I was so excited she felt up to undertaking the project. Although we had to postpone a days shooting because she had to fly to Houston for her chemical treatments, the very next day she was there all smiles and a new hairdo! She knew then, and wanted to have this last chance for everyone, especially her three young sons, to remember her looking as beautiful as she was. (Each time I watch the video, her radiance shines and tears of happiness brim my eyes. I thank God for being her friend.)

The video came out August 1, and Lauri entered the hospital that same month, never to return home again. She never got to see herself on national television or read the wonderful things said about her and our successful project, but when I'd visit her we'd talk about where I had been and what ladies everywhere were saying about the beautiful blonde chick in the video! Lauri said next time she wanted a speaking role.

It was a blessing on December 16, when God allowed her spirit to join him, leaving behind all the immense pain and suffering she went through during those last four

One Hundred Seventy-One

months. She had never complained; it was those around her who could not bear to see her suffer.

Thirty-four years is a very short time but I honestly believe Lauri lived a full life. She shared her joy, her love, her enthusiasm, her excitement, and most of all, her faith with everyone she came in contact with. This world and my life are both better, because Laurel Brumfield Richardson lived.

THE NIGHT THE BLUE LIGHT WENT OUT AT K-MART

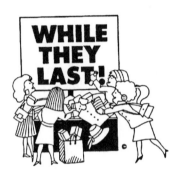

Chairman Joseph Antonini of the K-Mart chain today announced he is pulling the plug on the famous blue lights. Although the Blue Light Specials will continue, they will be without the flashing machine which drew customers to the designated marked downs. Instead the company will be installing a discount coupon machine to help consumers find current bargains. What is this world coming to?

Stores are becoming more and more complicated with their new lingo? Do you really understand the language? What is a price roll-back, anyway? Is that like a price markdown? Is it rolled up before it was rolled down? And every day low-price—is that today's price or yesterday's price or tomorrow's price? If it is a low price, does that mean it was once more than it is now, or are they planning to raise the price at a later date, thus making it a higher every day price then?

One Hundred Seventy-Three

Price slash sounds like it's unsafe to enter, doesn't it? I can conjure up mental images of half-crazed store clerks with straight razors ripping through the racks of leftovers. Price cut is a safer sounding, more gentle word. I don't like sales that seem dangerous or life threatening.

I sort of like those Two-for-One offers, but who ever needs two of whatever it is? If I didn't need one when it was at regular price, what are the chances I'll need two when it's on sale? (Still, I always seem to fall for this, and decide to give one as a gift. I have a whole hall closet full of future gifts that I can't seem to giveaway. When's your birthday?)

What ever happened to a good old fashioned sale? I used to love it on January 2nd and July 5th, when folks would line up outside the local clothing store cheering for the eight o'clock opening. It was a must to be there early to get the great bargains. People planned their vacations and even their operations around being on hand for these BIG shopping days. Women would push and shove and yell at each other as they all tried to grab up the perfect deal. Many a friendship has been destroyed during one of these wild events if only one size 12 blue dress could be found.

Those were the good ole days, before SPECIAL PURCHASE, Today's Special, Buy One-Get One Free, and 20% off every weekend started becoming the norm in America's retail. This was back when merchants didn't have to mark something up four times so they could make it half-price the next day. People appreciated merchandise, service, and loyalty.

Today is the first day of a new year, a better year so all the economic indicators predict. It's time to loosen up the purse strings and go shopping! I just received a mystery discount coupon letter from a new store down at the mall, I figure with my birthday discount, my husbands AARP card, my mall membership, and because it's raining on

Tuesday, I'll be able to purchase a dress, and the store will OWE me!

Thank God, I'm out of retail!

Yes, I am out of retail. I think I finally qualify as a writer now. Jojo would probably be extremely proud if she were here today to read this book that she inspired in her favorite grandchild. My first book, *WHAT MOTHER NEVER TOLD YA ABOUT RETAIL*, I did as an educational lesson, and as a tribute to the wonderful world of fashion retail. The video, ACCESSORY ADVANTAGE, I did as a sales tool and instructional guide for women everywhere who love accessorizing. (Both won first place awards from The National Federation of Press Women, as well as rave reviews.) This book, I did for the fun of it; I opened my heart and the words just poured out. (I got my awards up front in satisfaction.)

I think I managed to include everyone in my life on these pages from my husband and children, to Tom Cruise and Tom Landry. (By the way, I saw Tom #1 in "THE FIRM" this week. He's doing quite well for himself lately, and still looks as great as ever! Tom #2 this week agreed to be inducted into the Cowboy Ring of Fame in Texas Stadium. (I hope this doesn't mean I have to forgive Jerry Jones.)

My editor says it's five minutes to press time, and I'm still ramblin' on. What wonderful words of wisdom can I leave you with?

LOVE IS THE ANSWER, who cares what the question is?

No, that's too serious and romantic. How 'bout my motto:

"IT AINT OVER 'TIL THE FAT LADY SINGS"... And I don't even hear her warming up!

In CONCLUSION

There really is no ending to this section. The days go by and I continue to record my feelings about the world in general, and my life in particular, but I must stop somewhere. I have attempted to reveal to you the way I feel about the three F's: Fashion, Fun, and Feelings. (Perhaps, I should have added Food and Family to round off the title)

FASHION

I can't even imagine existing without fashion. It's always been such a thrill to wake up each morning and muse, "What'll I wear today?" Mixing, matching, and putting it all together has not only been a career and a challenge, but a way of life. Every little girl of my generation grew up playing paper dolls; I was born too early to experience the fun of Barbie. While most of these children were idolizing the beautiful models sweeping down the runways, I was admiring Edith Head, the lady whose talents designed most of the garments seen in the 1950's and 1960's Hollywood films. I dreamed of growing up to pursue a career in the glamorous world of fashion, and was able to make that dream come true.

FUN

How can I define such a word? If I asked a hundred different women, I'd get a hundred answers as to what it means to each individual. For me it's writing, reading, drawing, dreaming. It's travel, fancy earrings, family, shopping, friends, movies, books, and television.

One Hundred Seventy-Seven

For my mother, it's cooking, baking, planting flowers and working in her yard. Every woman of every generation has her own way of spelling F-U-N! And speaking of spelling, I even adore filling in the blanks on WHEEL OF FORTUNE and trying my hand at JEOPARDY.

Fun is sand between my toes, walking on the beach, reading U.S.A. TODAY without interruption! It's wearing yellow shoes, dreaming of Tom Cruise, and downing a peanut butter and jelly sandwich with a Diet Coke!

FEELINGS

This is the part where each of us really has a different outlook on life, molded by different upbringing, ruled by different emotions, and influenced by different memories. As I expressed mine, the thoughts and remembrances flowed onto the pages, yet I held millions deep inside of my heart. There are some things too precious to share and too hard to reveal in words.

How can I describe the heartbreaking sorrow of losing a child, except to say that God blessed me with my precious Laura Lea a year later? No words can explain the pride I feel for the son who has followed me into the garment trade, except to remind you: He is more handsome than Tom Cruise! And did I tell you how lucky I am to have a spider sitting on my shoulder each day, and sharing my life for the past twenty-five years?

Charles Swindoll wrote, *"The longer I live, the more I realize the impact of attitudes on life. Attitude, to me, is more important than facts. It is more important than circumstances, than money, than failures, than successes, than appearance, giftedness, or skill... The remarkable thing is we have a choice every day regarding the attitude we will embrace for the day. The only thing we can do is play on the one string we have, and that is our attitude... I am convinced that life is 10% what happens to me, and 90% how I react to it. And so it is with you, we are in charge of our attitudes."*

FASHION, FUN, and FEELINGS could have been named GARMENTS, GOOD TIMES, and *GOODBYES*. It was almost titled, *LOOKING AT LIFE*, or many other things I thought of during the months and years I worked on putting this together. In the end, I decided it is *A LADY LOOKS AT LIFE*.

Hopefully, my story will encourage you to take a look at your life and those who share it with you. Stop planning and wishing on hopes and dreams of tomorrow, and remember: THIS IS NOT A DRESS REHEARSAL. Take time to enjoy your *fashion, fun,* and *feelings* today!

One Hundred Eighty

OTHER PRODUCTS AVAILABLE BY T.J. REID

*WHAT MOTHER NEVER TOLD YA ABOUT
RETAIL*...a small store survival guide $29.95

*ACCESSORY ADVANTAGE: TACKY TO
TERRIFIC IN 10 EASY STEPS* , the video..............................$24.95

THE ACCESSORY ADVANTAGE HANDBOOK ....$ 5.00

THE EARRING SURVIVAL GUIDE ....$ 5.00

THE ACCESSORY SURVIVAL GUIDE ....$ 5.00

THE ACCESSORY SURVIVAL GUIDE PLUS...for
the Something More Woman ....$ 5.00

ACCESSORY ITEMS:

SLEEVEBANDS (page 39) Gold or Silver ....$ 6.00

STA-SCARF PIN (page 30) Gold or Silver ....$ 6.00

LARGE JEWELRY BAG (page 25) b/w dot $18.00

LARGE JEWERLY HANG-UP (page 26).............................$18.00

SCARF HANGER (page 29)..$ 6.00

TOTAL ....

Please send check or money order with full amount
including tax if you are a Louisiana resident to:

**T.J.'s...For Her, Inc.
P. O. Box 977
Amite, Louisiana 70422
504-748-8615
504-748-8930 Fax**

For information on any of the above products or T.J.
Reid's speaking schedule and availability, please contact
the above phone number or Fax.

One Hundred Eighty-One